Allergies to Milk

Allergies to Milk

Sami L. Bahna, M.D., Dr.P.H.

Assistant Professor of Pediatrics
Louisiana State University School of Medicine
Director, Division of Allergy and Immunology
Department of Pediatrics
Louisiana State University Medical Center
New Orleans, Louisiana

Douglas C. Heiner, M.D., Ph.D.

Professor of Pediatrics
University of California School of Medicine
Los Angeles, California
Chief, Division of Immunology and Allergy
Department of Pediatrics
Harbor-UCLA Medical Center
Torrance, California

GRUNE & STRATTON
A Subsidiary of Harcourt Brace Jovanovich, Publishers
NEW YORK   LONDON   TORONTO   SYDNEY   SAN FRANCISCO

Library of Congress Cataloging in Publication Data

Bahna, Sami L
 Allergies to milk.

 Bibliography: p.
 Includes index.
 1. Food allergy in children. 2. Milk as food. 3. Infants—Diseases. I. Heiner, Douglas C., joint author. II. Title.
 [DNLM: 1. Food hypersensitivity. 2. Milk—Adverse effects. WS310 B151a]
 RJ386.5.B33   618.92'975   80-13687
 ISBN 0-8089-1256-9

© 1980 by Grune & Stratton, Inc.
All rights reserved. No part of this publication
may be reproduced or transmitted in any form or
by any means, electronic or mechanical, including
photocopy, recording or any information storage
and retrieval system, without permission in
writing from the publisher.

Grune & Stratton, Inc.
111 Fifth Avenue
New York, New York 10003

Distributed in the United Kingdom by
Academic Press, Inc. (London) Ltd.
24/28 Oval Road, London NW 1

Library of Congress Catalog Number 80-13687
International Standard Book Number 0-8089-1256-9

Printed in the United States of America

To our wives
Reidun and Joy

>who have encouraged and assisted us
in the preparation of this manuscript
and who, incidentally, breastfed each
of their children six months or
more (ten children in all).

Contents

Foreword   *John W. Gerrard, D.M.*   x
Preface   xi
Acknowledgments   xii

Chapter 1
Introduction and Historical Background   1

Chapter 2
Epidemiology   5
    Evolution of the problem
    Prevalence
    Age at onset
    Sex distribution

Chapter 3
Composition of Cow's Milk   11
    Nutritional constituents of cow's milk
    Commercial forms of cow's milk
    Allergens in cow's milk
    Cross-reactivity of cow's milk proteins
    Foreign substances in cow's milk
    Effect of processing

Chapter 4
Pathogenesis 23
  Immune responses to cow's milk proteins in healthy persons
  Immune responses to cow's milk proteins in milk-sensitive patients
  Intrauterine sensitization
  Role of gastrointestinal tract
  Role of secretory IgA
  Immunologic mechanisms

Chapter 5
Manifestations 45
  Gastrointestinal manifestations
  Respiratory manifestations
  Dermatologic manifestations
  Hematologic manifestations
  Central nervous system manifestations
  Urinary manifestations
  Cardiovascular manifestations
  Miscellaneous manifestations

Chapter 6
Diagnosis 83
  History and clinical picture
  Challenge tests
  Skin tests
  In vitro tests

Chapter 7
Differential Diagnosis 109
  Other allergens
  Allergy to foreign substances in cow's milk
  Gastrointestinal disorders
  Respiratory disorders
  Dermatologic disorders

Chapter 8
Management 123
  Dietary management
  Pharmacologic agents
  Hyposensitization

Chapter 9
Prognosis 137

Chapter 10
Prevention 141
  Breast-feeding
  Other milk substitutes
  Introduction of other foods
  Role of the medical profession
  Role of women's organizations
  Role of infant–food industry

Appendix A.
Milk-Free Recipes 175

Appendix B.
Reference Tables on the Composition of Human Milk, Cow's Milk, Goat's Milk, and a Variety of Proprietary Formulas 189

Index 197

Foreword

Clinicians, while well equipped to handle diseases manifested by their patients, would much prefer to see these same diseases referred to as historical curiosities. Smallpox in our time has become such a curiosity, diphtheria in many quarters is almost so, and poliomyelitis, which not so long ago hung as a crippling spector over the strongest of our children, no longer haunts us. Rh disease, phenylketonuria, galactosemia, and congenital hypothyroidism are joining their ranks. As one disease after another is recognized, conquered and eliminated, attention is focused on those that remain. Among these are certain common respiratory and gastrointestinal problems that have not appeared to fit into the general tapestry of childhood disease. Children with these problems often have a persistent rhinorrhea or repeated attacks of bronchopneumonia, recurrent bouts of diarrhea, and vomiting with no clear-cut pathology, or fail to thrive for no tangible reason, and then just as all hope has been given up at discovering the cause of their illness—and sometimes just when a definitive diagnosis has been reached— they have again surprised us and have recovered. It is among these babies that those with allergies to cow's milk are found. Some are quickly recognized and shrewdly handled by the practicing physician. Others, with more complicated features, often gravitate to hospitals where they have presented perplexing problems in diagnosis and management.

The authors of this book have done a great service not only to physicians but also to their patients by bringing together in one volume a well documented review of the manifestations, epidemiology, pathology, immunology, management, and prognosis of patients with allergies to milk. Their objective approach brings much needed credibility to a subject that has at times spiked controversy. As the profession comes to appreciate fully the protean manifestations of milk allergy and then realizes that identical reactions can be triggered by other foods, a more rational approach to management of this group of disorders will materialize, and the subject will receive the treatment it deserves in standard text.

Drs. Bahna and Heiner conclude their volume by drawing attention to the overall importance of breast-feeding, both to the child and to the mother, and by emphasizing its importance in the prevention of cow's milk allergy. If their recommendations are followed as closely as they would wish, cow's milk allergy in infants should in its turn become a historical curiosity.

John W. Gerrard, D.M., F.R.C.P.(C.)
Professor of Pediatrics
University of Saskatchewan
Saskatoon, Saskatchewan, Canada

Preface

Data on allergic reactions to milk have needed compilation into one source for two reasons. First, a large volume of data has accumulated over almost a century. Second, clinicians earnestly trying to help their patients have taken divergent attitudes toward milk allergy, which frequently results in its underdiagnosis by some and its overdiagnosis by others. Hence health professionals need factual knowledge of the findings and views of leading workers in the field.

It is with this goal in mind that this book was written. The book is directed to a variety of potential readers, including practitioners in various disciplines, researchers, nutritionists, nurses, medical students, and the interested general public. Meeting the needs of such a wide variety of readers necessitated our collecting data from many sources and presenting them in a cohesive form. In doing so, the emergence of our personal attitudes in some sections of the book was inevitable, as was the discussion of some controversial points. Perhaps such controversies will stimulate further research.

The task of writing the chapter *Pathogenesis,* in particular, was facilitated by the relevant work of many reserachers who appropriately applied the techniques available to them and meticulously recorded their observations. The reader will notice that the disturbing gap in understanding the immunologic mechanisms in milk allergy—as well as in food allergy in general—is now being bridged to some extent. Many points still await clarification.

The nonmedical reader will comprehend many parts of the book, particularly the chapters *Manifestations, Diagnosis, Prognosis, Management,* and *Prevention.* Easy to prepare milk-free recipes, often devoid of other common food allergens as well, are included in the appendix and should be of help to milk-sensitive patients.

Health professionals in the fields of obstetrics, pediatrics, family practice, and nutrition should find the chapter *Prevention* of value as they advise parents on proper infant feeding.

Finally, we hope this effort helps to accomplish the goals of minimizing the incidence of milk allergy, facilitating its early recognition, and providing appropriate management. Achieving those goals should result in less physical and emotional suffering, avoidance of unnecessary diagnostic and therapeutic procedures, and a reduction in the cost of medical care.

Acknowledgments

We are grateful to Mrs. Mary Sue Brantley for her untiring and skilled assistance, particularly in library search. We also acknowledge the expert editorial assistance of Miss Virginia Howard. Our thanks are due to several authors and publishers who kindly gave us the permission to reproduce their material. We are indebted to our families for bearing with us when we frequently secluded ourselves in preparing this endeavor.

1
Introduction and Historical Background

Until recently, allergy to cow's milk was a controversial subject toward which many physicians had differing attitudes. Some textbooks of pediatrics either avoid mentioning cow's milk allergy or only lightly refer to it in relation to gastrointestinal symptoms. A few clinicians do not believe the condition exists and thus are understandably reluctant to diagnose it. On the other hand, there are those, particularly among pediatricians and to a lesser extent among general practitioners, who overzealously label infants "milk-sensitive" and who are inclined to recommend discontinuing the use of cow's milk whenever an infant has a gastrointestinal upset, respiratory symptoms, or a skin rash. Among the reasons for such divergent attitudes are (1) the variety of symptoms caused by cow's milk allergy, many of which may also occur as manifestations of other morbid conditions, and (2) the lack of a reliable single practical laboratory diagnostic test. Public awareness of cow's milk allergy, though increasing, is still marginal. Parents frequently are incredulous that milk could cause the symptoms their infant is exhibiting. The prevailing attitude is that cow's milk is not only a desirable food, but the ideal food and an essential element of the child's diet.

Hippocrates (460-370 B.C.) was one of the first to record that cow's milk could cause gastric upset and urticaria.[1] Later, Galen (131-210 A.D.) described a case of allergy to goat's milk.[2] Although ruminant milk has probably been used as a food to some degree since man began to record his activities, in early times human breast milk was the major food available to infants. When the mother was unable to nurse her baby, a wet nurse was almost the only alternative. People seldom thought of giving the calf's food to their babies.

The demand for wet nurses grew considerably during the seventeenth and eighteenth centuries. Women of a high social level in European countries increasingly wanted to use surrogate breast-feeding, claiming that breast-feeding might ruin their figures or impair their health. As Wickes[3] implied, perhaps the greatest force behind the declining popularity of nursing among the well-to-do was that it interfered with the mother's participation in social activities. Animal milk for infant feeding rose in popularity about the middle of the eighteenth century, with a preference of ass's and goat's milk over cow's milk.

At the beginning ot the twentieth century, reports of milk allergy began to appear in the German medical literature.[4] In 1905, Schlossman[5] documented symptoms of acute shock after ingestion of cow's milk. In the same year, Finkelstein[6] reported a death attributed to cow's milk ingestion, and he was the first to suggest oral hyposensitization. In 1908, severe reactions to cow's milk were described in the French literature.[7] A report from Sweden on a case of idiosyncrasy to cow's milk appeared in 1910,[8] and one of the earliest American reports on cow's milk allergy was by Talbot, in 1916.[9] Reports in the British literature did not appear until the 1940s.[10] Since then, increasing numbers of physicians have become aware of the condition, and a spate of articles has been published confirming that cow's milk allergy is a real problem, that it can involve several systems of the human body, and that it may be manifest in a wide variety of symptoms and signs.

The literature shows some inconsistency in the terminology used to describe symptoms attributable to cow's milk ingestion. The terms *intolerance, sensitivity, hypersensitivity,* and *allergy* have sometimes been used interchangeably or as synonyms. The word *intolerance* (meaning "not able to endure") is a general term that in a strict sense describes any adverse reaction. We prefer to restrict its use to situations in which the underlying mechanism is nonimmunologic and to use the terms *hypersensitivity* and *allergy* when the evidence strongly suggests an immunologic cause. Untoward reactions to cow's milk may be related to diverse mechanisms including:

1. *Enzymatic,* such as lactase deficiency, which may be congenital, or even more commonly secondary to a variety of gastrointestinal diseases including cow's milk allergy. Another condition in which the ingestion of milk is deleterious, because of a specific enzyme deficiency, is galactosemia.
2. *Immunologic,* i.e., hypersensitivity reactions to cow's milk proteins. Reactions may occur either locally in the gastrointestinal tract or in a remote shock organ such as the respiratory tract or skin. The immunologic effect sometimes involves immediate-type hypersensitivity, Arthus-like responses, and occasionally cell-mediated reactions.

Frequently, in fact, multiple immune mechanisms are involved, as discussed in more detail in Chapter 4 (Pathogenesis). Thus, at present, a specific immunologic mechanism is not easily incriminated as the causative one because of the expertise and expense involved in identifying predominant mechanisms while excluding other potential contributing mechanisms.

REFERENCES

1. Chabot R: Pediatric Allergy. New York, McGraw-Hill, 1951
2. O'Keefe ES: The history of pediatric allergy, in Speer F (ed): The Allergic Child. New York, Harper & Row, 1963, p 3
3. Wickes IG: A history of infant feeding. II. Seventeenth and eighteenth centuries. Arch Dis Child 28:232–240, 1953
4. Hamburger F: Biologisches Uber die Eiweisskorper der Kuhmilch und Uber Sauglingsernahrung. Wien Klin Wochenschr 14:1202, 1901
5. Schlossman A: Ueber die Giftwirkung des Artfremden Eiweisses in der Milch auf den Organismus des Sauglings. Arch Kinderheilkd 41:99–103, 1905
6. Finkelstein H: Kuhmilch als Ursache akuter Ernahrungstorungen bei Sauglingen. Monatsschr Kinderheilkd 4:65–72, 1905
7. Hutinel V: Intolerance for milk and anaphylaxis in nurslings. La Clinique 15:227, 1908
8. Wernstedt W: The causes of inferiority of cow's milk as food for feeble children: Infantile idiosyncrasy to cow's milk. Hygeia 72:629–644, 1910
9. Talbot FB: Idiosyncrasy to cow's milk: Its relation to anaphylaxis. Boston Med Surg J 175:409–410, 1916
10. Brodribb HS: Allergic vomiting in infants. Arch Dis Child 19.140–142, 1944

2
Epidemiology

EVOLUTION OF THE PROBLEM

Allergy to cow's milk became a significant health problem with the beginning of the twentieth century, when the mass production of infant formulas was introduced. At that time, formulas were intended to be used when breast-feeding could not be provided. Unfortunately, such appropriate logic has become diffused and is seldom considered by the average mother of today. For a variety of reasons, the use of cow's milk formula in infant feeding now prevails to the extent that most infants, particularly in industrialized countries, never even taste the food that has been created solely for them. The use of cow's milk formulas in infant feeding was introduced at a fortunate time for the dairy industry; today a study proposing the feeding of cow's milk to newborn infants would probably not be approved by a "Committee on human investigation." Three decades ago in the United States, about 65 percent of parturient mothers breast-fed their babies in the hospital.[1] In the early 1970s, 28 percent of 1-week-old infants were being breast-fed; the percentage declined to 15 percent for infants 2 months old.[2] Breast-feeding was even less prevalent among the lower socioeconomic groups than among those with higher income. In England, the percentage of breast-fed infants dropped from 60 percent in 1948 to about 40 percent in 1968.[3] In Canada, the prevalence of breast-feeding in 1973 was 35 percent during the first week of life, 17 percent at 3 months, and 6 percent at 6 months of age.[4]

Along with this decrease in breast-feeding, the number of morbid conditions in formula-fed infants increased.[5] Allergists and pediatricians have been long aware of a rising incidence of allergic disorders during infancy, the age in which foods are the most common allergens, with cow's milk on the top of the list of offenders.[6-9] Indeed, cow's milk sensitivity was noted in 30 percent of 109 allergic children under 2 years old.[10] The fact perhaps should not be surprising, for two reasons. First, cow's milk contains more than 25 distinct proteins that can be antigenic to infants who drink it. Second, cow's milk has become a commonplace in the daily diet of persons of all ages. In some societies, it quantitatively exceeds any other constituent of the diet, and in many others, its use is exceeded only by bread or rice.

PREVALENCE

Figures on the prevalence of cow's milk allergy vary widely from one study to another, because they are influenced by the following factors:

1. *Population studied.* A higher prevalence would be expected among sick subjects, particularly among those examined at an allergy clinic, than in the general population.
2. *Nature of infant feeding.* A higher prevalence might be expected in infants fed cow's milk from birth than in those who start cow's milk feedings later in life.[11, 12] The overall prevalence of cow's milk allergy is probably much less in societies in which breast-feeding still prevails.
3. *Age.* Cow's milk allergy is largely a disease of infancy, and its prevalence declines significantly beyond the age of 2 or 3 years.[13, 14]
4. *Investigator's attitude.* Cow's milk allergy is more likely to be diagnosed by investigators who are convinced of its occurrence than by those who are more skeptical of its existence.
5. *Diagnostic criteria.* Cow's milk allergy is overdiagnosed when the diagnosis depends exclusively on symptoms disappearing after a single trial of eliminating milk from the diet. On the other hand, relying on a particular laboratory finding is at present too strict a criterion and would exclude many true cases of cow's milk allergy. The same can be said of requiring symptoms to clear after milk has been eliminated and to recur on milk challenge at three separate occasions. Goldman et al.[15] noted that only 12.7 percent of children who were suspected of having milk allergy could meet such criteria.
6. *Type of study.* Figures derived from prospective studies are more reliable than those from retrospective studies in which the diagnoses were made by different physicians without preset criteria.
7. *Duration of study.* The longer the duration of follow-up and the more frequent and detailed the examination, the more subjects will be discovered who have symptoms that might be attributed to allergy.

Reported prevalence of cow's milk allergy varies between 0.3 and 7.5 percent (Table 2-1). Perhaps the true prevalence in the general pediatric popula-

Epidemiology

Table 2-1
Reported Prevalence of Cow's Milk Allergy

Author	Prevalence %	Population
Loveless[17]	1.5	Pediatric and adults
Clein[18]	6–8	Artificially fed infants
Collins-Williams[19]	0.3	Nonallergic under 15 yr, private practice
Glaser[20]	7	Private pediatric practice
Bachman and Dees[21]	1	Well babies under 2 yr
Fries[22]	< 3	Private pediatric practice
Freier and Kletter[23]	0.5	Well babies under 2 yr
Gerrard et al.[24]	7.5	Newborns followed 12–36 mo
Halpern et al.[12]	0.9	7–84 mo, no cow's milk in 1st 6 mo
Halpern et al.[12]	1.8	0–84 mo, on cow's milk in 1st 6 mo

Modified with permission from Bahna SL, Heiner DC: Cow's milk allergy: pathogenesis, manifestations, diagnosis and management, in Barness LA, et al. (eds): Advances in Pediatrics, vol. 25. Chicago, Year Book, 1978, pp 1–37.

tion of Western countries is somewhere between 1 and 3 percent. Accordingly, in the United States, where over 3 million infants are born per year, under the current practices of infant feeding 30 to 90 thousand new infants each year would be expected to suffer from cow's milk allergy.

AGE AT ONSET

Cow's milk allergy, mainly a disease of infancy, is usually manifested within the first 2 or 3 months of life.[14, 25, 26] Goldman et al.[15] studied 89 milk-sensitive children under 12 years of age and found that in 52 (58 percent) the age at onset of symptoms was under one month. Kuitunen et al.[27] reported the onset of symptoms at ages ranging from 1 day to 22 weeks, with a mean of 9 weeks. In the series of Gerrard et al.,[24] symptoms in 41 percent of milk-sensitive infants appeared within 7 days of starting cow's milk formula and in 69 percent within 4 weeks. No age, however, is exempt, and milk allergy may be first detected during adolescence or adulthood.[17, 28-31]

SEX DISTRIBUTION

Table 2-2 shows the number of males and females with cow's milk allergy as noted in various studies. The sex distribution appears to be equal except during early infancy, when more males seem to be affected, a tendency that is simlar to that of allergic disorders in general during early childhood.[12, 37]

Table 2-2
Sex Distribution of Patients with Cow's Milk Allergy

Author	No. of Males	No. of Females	Age
Gryboski[14]	18	3	2 d– 4 mo*
Gerrard et al.[24]	33	26	12– 36 mo
Matthews and Soothill[25]	6	2	10 d– 4 mo*
Kuitunen et al.[27]	25	29	4 d– 44 wk
Matsumura et al.[29]	14	10	6 mo– 31 yr
Liu et al.[31]	3	4	6 mo– 52 yr
Gamo et al.[32]	4	2	4– 29 mo
Boat et al.[33]	3	3	7– 48 mo
Fontaine and Navarro[34]	12	19	3– 20 mo
Harris et al.[35]	9	5	Under 1 yr*
Walker-Smith[36]	21	19	Children

*Remarkable male preponderance.

REFERENCES

1. Bain K: The incidence of breast-feeding in hospitals in the United States. Pediatrics 2:313– 319, 1948.
2. Fomon SJ: Infant Nutrition (ed 2). Philadelphia, Saunders 1974, p 8
3. Vahlquist B: Amningssituationen i i- och u-land: Tid for omvardering: Semper Nutrition Symposium. Naringsforskning 17 (Suppl 8):17, 1973
4. American Academy of Pediatrics, Committee on Nutrition: Breast-feeding. Pediatrics 62: 591– 601, 1978
5. Jelliffe EPP: Infant feeding practices: Associated iatrogenic and commerciogenic diseases. Pediatr Clin North Am 24:49– 61, 1977
6. Gerrard JW: Allergy in infancy. Pedatr Ann 3:9– 23, 1974
7. Matsumura T, Kuroume T, Tajima S: Acetonemic vomiting from viewpoint of food allergy. Acta Allergol (Kbh) 25:423– 450, 1970
8. Speer F: Multiple food allergy. Ann Allergy 34:71– 76, 1975
9. Speer F: Food allergy: The 10 common offenders. Am Fam Physician 13:106– 112, 1976
10. Bachman KD, Dees SC: Milk Allergy. II. Observations on incidence and symptoms of allergy in all allergic infants. Pediatrics 20:400– 407, 1957
11. Glaser J, Johnstone DE: Prophylaxis of allergic disease in newborn. JAMA 153:620– 622, 1953
12. Halpern SR, Sellars WA, Johnson RB, et al.: Development of childhood allergy in infants fed breast, soy or cow milk. J Allergy Clin Immunol 51:139– 151, 1973
13. Clein NW: Cow's milk allergy in infants and children. Int Arch Allergy Appl Immunol 13:245– 256, 1958
14. Gryboski JD: Gastrointestinal milk allergy in infants. Pediatrics 40:354– 362, 1967
15. Goldman AS, Anderson DW, Jr, Sellers WA, et al.: Milk allergy. I. Oral challenge with milk and isolated milk proteins in allergic children. Pediatrics 32:425– 443, 1963

Epidemiology

16. Bahna SL, Heiner DC: Cow's milk allergy: Pathogenesis, manifestations, diagnosis and management, in Barness LA, et al. (eds): Advances in Pediatrics, vol. 25. Chicago, Year Book, 1978, pp 1–37
17. Loveless MH: Milk allergy: A survey of its incidence; experiments with a masked ingestion test. J Allergy 21:489–499, 1950
18. Clein NW: Cow's milk allergy in infants. Pediatr Clin North Am 4:949–962, 1954
19. Collins-Williams C: The incidence of milk allergy in pediatric practice. J Pediatr 48:39–47, 1956
20. Glaser J: Allergy in Childhood. Springfield, Ill., Thomas, 1956, pp 441–462
21. Bachman KD, Dees SC: Milk allergy. I. Observations on incidence and symptoms in "well" babies. Pediatrics 20:393–399, 1957
22. Fries JH: Milk allergy: Diagnostic aspects and the role of milk substitutes. JAMA 165:1542–1545, 1957
23. Freier S, Kletter B: Milk allergy in infants and young children. Clin Pediatr 9:449–454, 1970
24. Gerrard JW, Mackenzie JWA, Goluboff N, et al.: Cow's milk allergy: Prevalence and manifestations in an unselected series of newborns. Acta Paediatr Scand Suppl 234:1–21, 1973
25. Matthews TS, Soothill JF: Complement activation after milk feeding in children with cow's milk allergy. Lancet 2:893–895, 1970
26. Lebenthal E: Cow's milk protein allergy. Pediatr Clin North Am 22:827–833, 1975
27. Kuitunen P, Visakorpi JK, Savilahti E, et al.: Malabsorption syndrome with cow's milk intolerance. Arch Dis Child 50:351–356, 1975
28. Pock-Steen OC, Niordson A-M: Milk Sensitivity in dermatitis herpetiformis. Br J Dermatol 83:614–619, 1970
29. Matsumura T, Kuroume T, Amada K: Close relationship between lactose intolerance and allergy to milk protein. J Asthma Res 9:13–19, 1971
30. Rapp DJ: Milk allergy from birth to old age. Consultant 14:120–122, 1974
31. Liu H-Y, Whitehouse WM, Giday Z: Proximal small bowel transit pattern in patients with malabsorption induced by bovine milk protein ingestion. Pediatr Radiol 115:415–420, 1975
32. Gamo I, Nishida M, Ikeda T, et al.: Studies on the antigenicity of cow's milk in infants. Med J Osaka Univ 18:397–415, 1968
33. Boat TF, Polmar SH, Whitman V, et al.: Hyperreactivity to cow's milk in young children with pulmonary hemosiderosis and cor pulmonale secondary to nasopharyngeal obstruction. J Pediatr 87:23–29, 1975
34. Fontaine JL, Navarro J: Small intestinal biopsy in cow's milk protein allergy in infancy. Arch Dis Child 50:357–362, 1975
35. Harris MJ, Petts V, Penny R: Cow's milk allergy as a cause of infantile colic: Immunofluorescent studies on jejunal mucosa. Aust Paediatr J 13:276–281, 1977
36. Walker-Smith JA: Gastrointestinal allergy. Practitioner 220:562–573, 1978
37. Bahna SL: A statistical study of allergic disorders among school children. Thesis for Doctorate Degree in Public Health, University of Alexandria, Egypt, 1970

3
Composition of Cow's Milk

NUTRITIONAL CONSTITUENTS OF COW'S MILK

Cow's milk is considered a good source of high-quality protein, fat, carbohydrate, vitamins A and B, and minerals (Appendix B, Tables 1 to 3). All essential amino acids are present in adequate quantities. Milk is deficient, however, in iron and vitamins C and D. In many countries, marketed pasteurized milk is usually fortified with 400 IU of vitamin D per liter. Adequate supplements of vitamins and sometimes of iron too are added to proprietary cow's milk formulas.

Protein

On the average, pooled whole cow's milk contains 3.3 gm protein/dl, with a ragne of 2.8 to 4.1 gm/dl (Table 3-1). The two main components of cow's milk protein are casein, which constitutes about 80 percent, and whey proteins, which constitute about 20 percent. Individual protein constitutents vary quantitatively with the stage of lactation, the breed of cattle, and the feed used, apparently with little qualitative variation.[2]

Bovine caseins exist as a colloidal complex with calcium phosphate.[3] In order of decreasing electrophoretic mobility at alkaline pH, the four major caseins are called alpha, beta, gamma, and kappa caseins and have molecular weights ranging between 18,000 and 24, 000 daltons.[4] Beta-lactoglobulin is the major whey protein and is composed of two identical polypeptide chains, each having a molecular weight of about 18,000 daltons. The term *lactalbumin* may be misleading, because this whey protein fraction contains a heterogeneous group of

Table 3-1
Bovine Milk Proteins

Protein Fractions	Molecular Weight	mg/100 ml Skim Milk	Percent
Caseins			
$\alpha,\beta,\gamma,\kappa$	18,000–24,000	2500–2800	76–86
Whey Proteins		350–650	14–24
Lactalbumin fraction		300–450	10–16
β-lactoglobulin	18,000	200–300	7–12
α-lactalbumin	15,000	70–100	2–5
Serum albumin	68,000	30–40	0.7–1.3
Immunoglobulins		50–100	1.4–2.8
IgG	150,000–170,000	50–85	1.2–2.5
IgM	900,000–1,000,000	5–10	0.1–0.2
IgA	300,000–500,000	2–5	0.05–0.1

From Bahna SL: Control of milk allergy: A challenge for physicians, mothers and industry. Ann Allergy 41:1–12, 1978

proteins that are soluble in saturated ammonium sulfate. Bovine alpha-lactalbumin is a protein of a single polypeptide chain with a molecular weight of about 15,000 daltons. Serum albumin also is composed of a single polypeptide chain and has a molecular weight of about 68,000 daltons. Immunoglobulins constitute about 2 percent of the total bovine milk proteins (more in colostrum), with IgG being the most, IgM intermediate, and IgA the least in quantity. Both casein and beta-lactoglobulin are synthesized locally by the mammary gland from amino acids supplied by the blood, and they have no obvious relationship to any of the plasma proteins.[4] Beta-lactoglobulin, though considered a pure protein, showed heterogenicity when preparations from different cows were compared. Three genetic variants of bovine beta-lactoglobulin have been identified by starch-gel electrophoresis, and were designated as A, B, and C, according to their speed of mobility. An individual cow may produce any of the three variants singly or together with either of the other two variants. Immunologically, however, all three variants were found to be identical.[5]

Carbohydrate

Lactose is the only carbohydrate and is present in quantities ranging between 4.5 and 5.0 gm/dl, with an average of 4.8 gm/dl.

Fat

The fat content ranges between 3.1 and 5.2 gm/dl (a mean of 3.7 gm/dl), and is more variable than any other constituent. Cream is composed principally of the triglycerides olein, palmitin, and stearin, and, to a lesser extent, cholesterol. The cholesterol content of whole cow's milk is 9 to 17 mg/dl, and in skim

Composition of Cow's Milk

milk only 0.4 mg/dl. The content of saturated fatty acids is about 2.5 times that of polyunsaturated fat.

Calories

Whole cow's milk provides 20 calories per ounce, 50 percent derived from fat, 30 percent from carbohydrate, and 20 percent from protein.

More details about the biochemistry of bovine milk are available from several sources.[6-10]

COMMERCIAL FORMS OF COW'S MILK

Milk in its raw form is not recommended for feeding, and its sale is forbidden in most countries. *Pasteurization* destroys pathogenic bacteria in milk and modifies its casein so that less tough curds are formed in the stomach. Accepted pasteurization temperatures are either 63°C for 30 minutes, or, as is more commonly used, 72°C for 15 seconds. Pasteurized milk should be kept refrigerated, and boiling is recommended before it is fed to infants. Homogenization is accomplished by breaking fat globules into a homogeneous emulsion of minute particles that no longer separate on standing.

Condensed milk has a high sugar content (approximately 60 percent) through the addition of sucrose. It is used in dilutions 1:10 to 1:4 to provide a formula high in sugar and low in fat and protein. It is not used in routine infant feeding except for short periods when a high caloric intake is required.

Skim milk is available either as half-skim milk (1.5 gm fat/dl) or nonfat skim milk (0.05 gm fat/dl).

Evaporated milk has a water content of 73 to 74 percent compared with 83 to 88 percent for whole milk, and the casein curd formed in the stomach is softer. It has 44 calories per ounce and is diluted with an equal quantity of water before feeding.

A wide variety of *standard cow's milk formulas* are commercially available in various countries. Examples and composition of such formulas are presented in Appendix B, Table 4. Generally, they are modified to resemble the nutritional composition of human milk, most of them are supplemented with vitamins, and many are fortified with iron. The titrable acidity of many cow's milk formulas is much higher than that of human milk, and their osmolality may vary between 193 and 381 mOsm/Kg water.[10a] Formulas with low acid load and of low osmolality should be preferred, particularly in sick infants.

ALLERGENS IN COW'S MILK

Although intolerance to cow's milk may be caused by a wide variety of inherited or acquired defects in the digestion or absorption of its carbohydrate, fat, or protein, hypersensitivity reactions are largely attributable to the protein components. Neither milk fat nor lactose itself has been shown to be antigenic. Commercial preparations of lactose, however, may be contaminated with bovine milk proteins. Hence, caution must be exercised in attributing allergy symptoms to ingested lactose. Spies[11] reported that the commercial lactose he studied contained small amounts of known milk proteins as well as four antigens that were distinct from the known milk proteins. No evidence was presented, however, for the allergenicity of these unnamed antigens in man. The allergenicity of cow's milk proteins may possibly be enhanced by a Maillard (nonenzymatic) reaction with lactose, which results in N-glycosidic coupling of the sugar into the protein molecule.[10, 12-14] In atopic persons with milk hypersensitivity, the skin reactivity to beta-lactoglobulin was increased a hundredfold by prior reacting of the protein with lactose.[13]

Cow's milk contains more than 25 separate protein components that may induce specific antibody production in man.[15-18] Many bovine serum proteins have been shown by means of immunoelectrophoresis to be present in cow's milk.[16-19] Hinkle et al.[20] showed that bovine serum gamma globulin and serum albumin are frequently precipitated by human sera containing precipitins to cow's milk proteins. Therefore, the ingestion of cow's milk may be regarded as the ingestion of specific milk proteins manufactured in the mammary gland plus bovine serum proteins. Serum proteins in milk, though present in low concentrations, may be antigenic and may cause hypersensitivity reactions. For example, milk-induced gastrointestinal bleeding may increase when bovine serum albumin is used as the challenging antigen.[21] Because of the difficulty in isolating and preparing many immunologically pure serum or milk protein fractions, a precise evaluation of antigen-antibody reactions to cow's milk has been a problem. A number of studies have shed a great deal of light on the subject of serum antibodies to cow's milk proteins. All investigators agree that the allergenicities of various cow's milk proteins definitely differ.

Ratner et al.,[22] in studies of guinea pig anaphylaxis, found that beta-lactoglobulin was more allergenic than casein or alpha-lactalbumin. Parish,[23] using passive cutaneous anaphylaxis in monkeys, also noted that human antibodies were most frequently directed toward beta-lactoglobulin. In a group of milk-sensitive infants, serum IgE antibodies to different cow's milk protein fractions were studied and were found to be directed most frequently against beta-lactoglobulin.[24] Similar findings were noted in patients with cow's milk allergy when they were orally challenged with cow's milk protein fractions.[25-30]

In a series of 45 children with cow's milk allergy, Goldman et al.[25] noted a reaction after oral challenge: with beta-lactoglobulin, in 62 percent of the children; with casein, in 60 percent; with alpha-lactalbumin, in 53 percent; and with bovine serum albumin, in 52 percent; the resulting reactions were similar to those that occurred after challenges with skim milk. Lebenthal,[31] compiling the results of five studies,[25-29] noted that sensitivity to beta-lactoglobulin occurred in 82 percent of patients; to casein, in 43 percent; to alpha-lactalbumin, in 41 percent;

to bovine gamma globulin, in 27 percent; and to bovine serum albumin, in 18 percent. Skin-testing also showed that in both pasteurized and raw cow's milk the reactive component resided largely in the beta-lactoglobulin fraction.[13, 32] Nevertheless, in a study on a group of children, most of whom had respiratory illnesses, precipitins to bovine serum albumin and bovine gamma globulin were detected more frequently than precipitins to casein, beta-lactoglobulin, and alpha-lactalbumin.[33]

Because of the observation that the allergencity of beta-lactoglobulin may be potentiated by the browning reaction with lactose,[12] some workers have hypothesized that during digestion a milk protein antigen may react with a carbohydrate and become a more potent allergen.[14] The amount of antigen required to elicit a positive intradermal reaction in atopic persons fell from 10 mcg for crystalline beta-lactoglobulin to 0.1 μg for the beta-lactoglobulin-lactose preparation.[8, 12]

CROSS-REACTIVITY OF COW'S MILK PROTEINS

Goat's Milk.

Frequently goat's milk has been substituted for cow's milk in milk allergy. Hill[34] studied 45 infants with eczema whose skin tests were positive to bovine lactalbumin; tests with goat's lactalbumin showed positive responses in 25 and doubtful responses in 10, suggesting that cross-reactions are frequent.

Antigenic similarity between cow's and goat's milk proteins were demonstrated by Saperstein[35] in a variety of ways:

1. Antisera to bovine beta-lactoglobulin and alpha-lactalbumin produced positive precipitin tests with goat's whey protein.
2. Rabbits were sensitized with small amounts of cow's milk protein and did not produce detectable antibodies for several months. When goat's whey protein was injected into the rabbits, an anamnestic reaction resulted in an increased production of antibodies to cow's milk proteins.
3. Guinea pigs that had been passively sensitized to cow's milk proteins with a single intraperitoneal injection of specific antiserum developed anaphylaxis when challenged 24 to 48 hours later with an intravenous injection of goat's whey proteins.

Using the double-gel diffusion technique of Ouchterlony,[36] Crawford and Grogan[37] found that alpha-casein, beta-lactoglobulin, and alpha-lactalbumin in goat's milk are immunologically related to the corresponding bovine fractions, and in the case of casein the precipitin patterns were almost completely identical. Jeness et al.[38] noted that antibody to bovine beta-lactoglobulin could react with beta-lactoglobulin from milk of cow, water buffalo, goat, and sheep.

In clinical studies,[28,29] infants with cow's milk allergy frequently responded to challenge with goat's milk.

Sheep's Milk.

Bovine and sheep's beta-lactoglobulins have been tested by double diffusion in agar and by immunoelectrophoresis using antisera prepared in rabbit against both kinds of beta-lactoglobulin. Complete cross-reactions were noted between each of the beta-lactoglobulins and the two types of antisera.[5] Possibly the molecular structures of cow's and sheep's beta-lactoglobulin are so similar that the rabbit's body was incapable of detecting the difference and thus the antibodies produced were identical. The cross-antigenicity of beta-lactoglobulin seems to be shared among most ruminant milks.[38] We did not find clinical studies that indicated cross-allergenicity between cow's and sheep's milks.

Cow's Hair.

Cross-reactivity between cow's milk proteins and cow's hair was demonstrated clinically by Osvath et al.[39] In that study, 7 out of 10 children who suffered from asthma after ingestion of cow's milk developed bronchospasms after bronchial provocation tests with cow's hair. In this instance, serum proteins may be the responsible allergens because they are found in both cow's milk and cow's hair.

Human Milk.

Cow's milk proteins and human milk proteins apparently do not cross-react.[40-42] When rabbit antiserum is used, however, some human serum proteins have partial identity to and cross-reactivity with the corresponding bovine serum proteins that are in cow's milk.[17] The clinical importance, if any, of this cross-reactivity is yet to be clarified.

FOREIGN SUBSTANCES IN COW'S MILK

Adverse reactions related to the ingestion of cow's milk are occasionally caused by foreign substances in the milk rather than by milk constitutents themselves. Such substances may reach the milk through a variety of ways, such as passage from the circulation into the mammary gland, injection into or application onto the udder, and adulteration or contamination of the milk during handling or processing.

Potentially allergenic substances that have been found in raw cow's milk include penicillin, wheat, peanut, linseed, cottonseed, ragweed, primula veris, and bacteria.[43] DDT may be present, usually in negligible quantities.[44] Lead, however, was present in significant concentrations in some samples of homogenized milk, evaporated milk, and cow's milk formulas.[45]

Antiobiotics were frequent contaminants of cow's milk in the past. Bovine mastitis was treated mainly by intramammary injection of penicillin and, less frequently, by other antibiotics such as streptomycin and tetracyclines. In the early 1950s, three surveys were carried out in the United States to determine the antibiotic content of fluid market milk.[46] Penicillin was detected in 3.2 to 11.6 percent of samples tested, and was present in concentrations from 0.003 to 0.55 unit/ml. Bacitracin was detected in 1 percent, and streptomycin was present in only 1 out of 1,706 milk samples. Whereas streptomycin and oxytetracyclines are not potent antigens when taken orally, penicillin has been known to be a potent allergen, and in even minute quantities it may induce severe reactions in exquisitely penicillin-sensitive subjects. To prevent this potential hazard, the Food and Drug Adminsitration in 1953[47] required manufacturers of antibiotics for bovine mastitis to insert a statement in each package that milk from treated cattle should not be sold for human consumption unless it is obtained at least 3 days after medication has been stopped. Conceivably, penicillin might also be added by milk distributors to reduce the bacterial count, and the Food and Drug Administration has prohibited this act and considered it an adulteration. In spite of this regulation, however, hypersensitivity reactions to penicillin present in milk continued to be reported.[46,48-50] Wicher et al.[51] documented that a woman known to be sensitive to penicillin had a severe allergic reaction after she drank milk that was found to contain about 10 units/ml of penicillin.

An inadvertent intravenous infusion of 100 ml of pasteurized milk in a young adult with duodenal ulcer has been reported.[52] Features of generalized immediate hypersensitivity reaction, including urticaria, developed within 10 minutes. Whether the symptoms were caused by an IgE-mediated hypersensitivity reaction or by another mechanism was not documented. After recovery, the patient did not develop any symptoms from drinking milk.

EFFECT OF PROCESSING

Heat constitutes the main method of the processing of milk, i.e., through the pasteurization, boiling, evaporation, or preparation of powdered milk. Heating causes certain changes in milk proteins, including unfolding of polypeptide chains and rupture of disulfide linkages. Boiling of milk is known to reduce curd tension and may alter the physical properties of milk proteins.[53] Certain milk proteins are more affected than others, and are called heat-labile milk constituents. Heat lability may be judged by a variety of criteria, one of which is immunologic reactivity.

Ratner et al.[54] were able to sensitize guinea pigs by feeding them pasteurized skim milk, but not by feeding them heat-denatured milk. Several studies,[43,55,56] in which heated milk and commercial preparations of evaporated milk were used, showed that alpha-casein was heat-stable, in that its antigenicity was not decreased until it was exposed to temperatures exceeding 100°C. Alpha-lactalbumin was moderately heat-labile, its antigenicity being somewhat impaired at 60°C and almost completely destroyed by the process of making evaporated milk. Beta-lactoglobulin was intermediate, being only partially denatured at 100°C. The relative heat stability of beta-lactoglobulin may be related to the formation of a more stable compound with lactose.[12] Luz and Todd[57] noted that bovine serum albumin was among the most heat-labile of milk proteins, whereas at least some of the antigenicity of casein, beta-lactoglobulin, and alpha-lactalbumin was retained in evaporated milk. Hanson and Mansson,[16] using immune electrophoretic analysis, found that casein resisted a temperature of 120°C for 15 minutes and beta-lactoglobulin and alpha-lactalbumin resisted heating to 100°C, but bovine serum proteins were denatured at 70° to 80°C. Cole and Dees,[58] in a study of guinea pigs, noted that some antigenicity of the whey proteins was retained in heat-processed cow's milk, and that alpha-lactalbumin was more antigenic than beta-lactoglobulin.

Saperstein[35] tested different commercial evaporated milk formulas and demonstrated positive precipitin reactions using antigens from some preparations but not from others, indicating inconsistency in the denaturation of milk proteins. In the same study, it was found that after guinea pigs had been passively sensitized with antisera to alpha-lactalbumin or beta-lactoglobulin, they often developed anaphylactic shock when challenged intravenously with reconstituted evaporated milk, indicating that these proteins could retain some allergenicity in the evaporated milk.

When a variety of proprietary infant milk formulas were studied by precipitin test and passive cutaneous anaphylaxis, Saperstein and Anderson[59] found that the antigenic determinants of casein, alpha-lactalbumin, and beta-lactoglobulin were not inactivated by the heat applied during the manufacturing processes used. Bovine serum albumin was found to be immunologically inactive in canned liquid milk preparations but was active in powdered milk formulas. Bovine gamma globulin activity was detected only in fresh pasteurized and spray-dried milks that had been subjected to minimal heat in their preparation.

Using the dual-ingestion passive transfer test, Crawford[60] found that the heat-denaturation of milk in the liquid or powder form before ingestion greatly reduced the allergenicity of beta-lactoglobulin and alpha-lactalbumin but not of alpha-casein. The ingestion of pasteurized milk (skimmed or homogenized), on the other hand, resulted in frequent reactions at the sites passively sensitized to any of the three protein fractions, alpha-casein, beta-lactoglobulin, or alpha-lactalbumin.

Crawford and Grogan[37] conducted precipitation experiments using double-gel diffusion technique with rabbit antisera and noted that heat-denatured milks completely lost their reactivity with antisera against alpha-lactalbumin and that the reactivity to antisera against alpha-casein and beta-lactoglobulin was greatly reduced. On the other hand, Nagel et al.,[61] on studying a series of milk-sensitive patients who had positive skin reactions to raw cow's milk proteins, found that the skin responses were not significantly reduced when the patients were tested with heat-treated whole cow's milk, casein, beta-lactoglobulin, or alpha-lactalbumin.

Based on the above studies, "heat denaturation" of cow's milk does not imply nonallergenicity. Heated milk seems to be most useful in patients sensitive solely to the heat-labile protein fractions, such as bovine serum albumin or bovine gamma globulin, and to a lesser extent in patients sensitive to alpha-lactalbumin. The characteristics of the main milk protein fractions are summarized in Table 3-2.

Table 3-2
Characteristics of the Main Protein Fractions in Cow's Milk

Protein Fraction	Approximate Distribution %	Allergenicity	Stability at 100°C
Caseins	82	++	+++
β-lactoglobulin	10	+++	++
α-lactalbumin	4	++	+
Serum albumin	1	+	±
Immunoglobulins	2	+	−

The antigenicity of trypsin digests of bovine casein, as tested by passive cutaneous anaphylaxis in guinea pigs and precipitin inhibition tests, was noted to be significantly reduced compared with the antigenicity of nondigested casein.[62] This difference in antigenicity has been supported by the observation that sera of infants fed casein hydrolysate formula had low titers of hemagglutinins to casein compared with the titers of the sera of infants fed regular cow's milk formula.[63] Occasional patients, however, may possibly be allergic to digests of milk proteins rather than to the native protein molecules themselves.[64]

As early as 1911, *ultraviolet radiation* was noted to reduce the antigenic activity of proteins.[65] Gamma radiation was subsequently found to be more effective than ultraviolet radiation but much less effective than heat in denaturing proteins.[37, 53] Samples of raw skimmed milk treated with 5.58 and 9.30 megarad showed an antigenic activity similar to that of milk heated for 35 minutes at 77° and 89°C, respectively.[53]

REFERENCES

1. Bahna SL: Control of milk allergy: A challenge for physicians, mothers and industry. Ann Allergy 41:1–12, 1978
2. McMeekin TL: The Proteins: Chemistry, Biological Activity, and Methods, vol II. New York, Academic Press, 1954, pp 389–434
3. King TP: Chemical and biological properties of some atopic allergens. Adv Immunol 23:77–105, 1976
4. White A, Handler P, Smith EL: Principles of Biochemistry (ed 5). New York, McGraw-Hill, 1973, pp 924–925
5. Bell K, McKenzie HA: β-lactoglobulins. Nature (London) 204:1275–1279, 1964
6. Butler JA: Bovine immunoglobulins: A review. J Dairy Sci 52:1895, 1969
7. McKenzie HA: Milk Proteins. New York, Academic Press, 1970
8. Bleumink E: Food allergy: The chemical nature of the substances eliciting symptoms. World Rev Nutr Diet 12:505–570, 1970
9. Lyster RLJ: Review of the progress of dairy science. Section C. Chemistry of milk proteins. J Dairy Res 39:279–318, 1972
10. Smith G: Whey protein. Would Rev Nutr Diet 24:88–116, 1976
10a. Toh CC, Ho NK: pH, titrable acidity & osmolality of human breast milk & some infant formulae. J Singapore Pediatr Soc 20:88–92, 1978
11. Spies JR: New antigens in lactose (35546). Proc Soc Exp Biol Med 137:211–214, 1971
12. Bleumink E, Berrens L: Synthetic approaches to the biological activity of β-lactoglobulin in human allergy to cow's milk. Nature (London) 212:541–543, 1966
13. Bleumink E, Young E: Identification of the atopic allergen in cow's milk. Int Arch Allergy 34:521–543, 1968
14. Lietze A: Laboratory research in food allergy. I. Food allergens. J Asthma Res 7:25–40, 1969
15. Hanson LA, Johansson B: Immune electrophoretic analysis of bovine milk protein fractions. Experientia 15:377–379, 1959
16. Hanson LA, Mansson I: Immune electrophoretic studies of bovine milk and milk products. Acta Paediatr Scand 50:484–490, 1961
17. Heiner DC, Wilson JF, Lahey ME: Sensitivity to cow's milk. JAMA 189:563–567, 1964
18. Lowenstein H, Krasilnikoff PA, Bjerrum OJ, et al.: Occurrence of specific precipitins against bovine whey proteins in serum from children with gastrointestinal disorders. Int Arch Allergy Appl Immunol 55:514–525, 1977
19. Gugler E, Bein M, von Muralt G: Über immunoelektrophoretische Untersuchungen an Kuhmilchprotein. Schweiz Med Wochenschr 89:1172–1176, 1959
20. Hinkle NH, Hong R, West CD: Identification of the antigen and symptomatology of children with precipitins to milk. Am J Dis Child 102:449–452, 1961
21. Wilson JF, Lahey ME, Heiner DC: Studies on iron metabolism. V. Further observations on cow's milk-induced gastrointestinal bleeding in infants with iron-deficiency anemia. J Pediatr 84:335–344, 1974
22. Ratner B, Dworetzky M, Oguri S, et al.: Studies on the allergenicity of cow's milk. I. The allergenic properties of alpha-casein, beta-lactoglobulin and alpha-lactalbumin. Pediatrics 22:449–452, 1958
23. Parish WE: Detection of reaginic and short-term sensitizing anaphylactic or anaphylactoid antibodies to milk in sera of allergic and normal persons. Clin Allergy 1:369–380, 1971
24. Kletter B, Gery I, Freier S, et al.: Immunoglobulin E antibodies to milk proteins. Clin Allergy 1:249–255, 1971
25. Goldman AS, Anderson DW, Jr, Sellers WA, et al.: Milk allergy. I. Oral challenge with milk and isolated milk proteins in allergic children. Pediatrics 32:425–443, 1963

26. Davidson M, Burnstine RC, Kugler MM, et al.: Malabsorption defect induced by ingestion of beta lacto-globulin. J Pediatr 66:545–554, 1965
27. Visakorpi JK, Immonen P: Intolerance to cow's milk and wheat gluten in the primary malabsorption syndrome in infancy. Acta Paediatr Scand 56:49–56, 1967
28. Freier S, Kletter B, Gery I, et al.: Intolerance to milk protein. J Pediatr 75:623–631, 1969
29. Lebenthal E, Laor J, Lewitus Z, et al.: Gastrointestinal protein loss in allergy to cow's milk β-lactoglobulin. Israel J Med Sci 6:506–510, 1970
30. Kuitunen P, Visakorpi JK, Savilahti E, et al.: Malabsorption syndrome with cow's milk intolerance. Arch Dis Child 50:351–356, 1975
31. Lebenthal E: Cow's milk protein allergy. Pediatr Clin North Am 22:827–833, 1975
32. De la Reguera IG, Subirá ML, Oehling A: The role of sensitizing proteins in milk allergy. Allergol et Immunopathol 6:225–230, 1978
33. Holland NH, Hong R, Davis NC, et al.: Significance of precipitating antibodies to milk proteins in the serum of infants and children. J Pediatr 61:181–195, 1962
34. Hill LW: Infantile eczema with a special reference to the use of a milk-free diet. JAMA 96:1277–1280, 1931
35. Saperstein S: Antigenicity of the whey proteins in evaporated cow's milk and whole goat's milk. Ann Allergy 18:765–773, 1960
36. Ouchterlony O: Antigen-antibody reactions in gel. IV. Types of reactions in coordinated systems of diffusion. Acta Pathol Microbiol Scand 32:231–240, 1953
37. Crawford LV, Grogan FT: Allergenicity of cow's milk proteins. IV. Relationship of goat's milk proteins as studied by serum-agar precipitation. J Pediatr 59:347–350, 1961
38. Jeness R, Phillip NI, Kalan EB: Immunological comparison of beta-lactoglobulins. Fed Proc 26:340, 1967
39. Osvath P, Muranyi L, Endre L, et al.: Investigation of the cross reaction of cow's hair and milk antigen in bronchial provocation. Acta Allergol 27:355–363, 1972
40. Gunther M, Aschaffenburg R, Matthews RH, et al.: The level of antibodies to the proteins of cow's milk in the serum of normal human infants. Immunology 3:296–306, 1960
41. Heiner DC, Sears JW, Kniker WT: Multiple precipitins to cow's milk in chronic respiratory disease. Am J Dis Child 103:634–654, 1962
42. Bahna SL, Heiner DC: Cow's milk allergy: Pathogenesis, manifestations, diagnosis and management, in Barness LA, et al. (ed): Advances in Pediatrics, vol 25. Chicago, Year Book, 1978, pp 1–37
43. Collins-Williams C: Cow's milk allergy in infants and children. Int Arch Allergy 20:38–59, 1962
44. Knowles JA: Breast milk: A source of more than nutrition for the neonate. Clin Toxicol 7:69–82, 1974
45. Lamm S, Cole B, Glynn K, et al.: Lead content of milks fed to infants, 1971–1972. N Engl J Med 289:574–575, 1973
46. Welch H: Problems of antibiotics in food as the Food and Drug Adminsitration sees them. Am J Public Health 47:701–705, 1957
47. Federal Register 18:1077, 1953
48. Vickers HR, Bagratuni L, Alexander S: Dermatitis caused by penicillin in milk. Lancet 1:351–352, 1958
49. Siegel BB: Hidden contacts with penicillin. Bull WHO 21:703–713, 1959
50. Borrie P, Barrett J: Dermatitis caused by penicillin in bulked milk supplies. Br Med J 2:1267, 1961
51. Wicher K, Reisman RE, Arbesman CE: Allergic reaction to penicillin present in milk. JAMA 208:143–145, 1969
52. Wallace JR, Payne RW, Mack AJ: Inadvertent intravenous infusion of milk. Lancet 6:1264–1266, 1972

53. Kraybill HF, Read MS, Lindner RO, et al.: The effect of heat processing, gamma radiation and ultraviolet radiation on the anaphylactogenic properties of milk. J Allergy 30:342–352, 1959
54. Ratner B, Dworetzky M, Oguri S, et al.: Studies on the allergenicity of cow's milk. III. Effect of heat treatment on the allergenicity of milk and protein fractions from milk as tested in guinea-pigs by sensitization and challenge by the oral route. Pediatrics 22:653–658, 1958
55. Davies W: Cow's milk allergy in infancy. Arch Dis Child 33:265–268, 1958
56. Ratner B, Dworetzky M, Oguri S, et al.: Studies on the allergenicity of cow's milk. II. Effect of heat treatment on the allergenicity of milk and protein fractions from milk as tested in guinea-pigs by parenteral sensitization and challenge. Pediatrics 22:648–652, 1958
57. Luz AQ, Todd RH: Antigenicity of heated milk proteins. Am J Dis Child 108:479–486, 1964
58. Cole WQ, Dees SC: Allergenic properties of milk and milk proteins. J Pediatr 63:256–263, 1963
59. Saperstein S, Anderson DW: Antigenicity of milk proteins of prepared formulas measured by precipitin ring test and passive cutaneous anaphylaxis in the guinea pig. J Pediatr 61:196–204, 1962
60. Crawford LV: Allergenicity of cow's milk proteins. I. Effect of heat treatment on the allergenicity of protein fractions of milk as studied by the dual ingestion passive transfer test. Pediatrics 25:432–436, 1960
61. Nagel JE, Miller DL, Friday GA, et al.: Does heating really enhance the digestibility of milk or alter its antigenicity? Pediatr Res 7:337, 1973
62. Gamo I, Nashida M, Ikeda T, et al.: Studies on the antigenicity of cow's milk in infants. Med J. Osaka Univ 18:397–415, 1968
63. Eastham EJ, Lichauce T, Grady MI, et al.: Antigenicity of infant formulas: Role of immature intestine on protein permeability. J Pediatr 93:561–564, 1978
64. Haddad ZH, Kalra V, Verma S: IgE antibodies to peptic and peptic-tryptic digests of beta-lactoglobulin: Significance in food hypersensitivity. Ann Allergy 42:368–371, 1979
65. Doerr R, Maldovan J: Die Wirkung des Ultravioletten Lightes auf das Eiwein-antigen und zeinen antikörpes. Wein Klin Wochenschr 24:555–559, 1911

4
Pathogenesis

It is not yet possible to explain in detail the pathogenesis of the diverse types of food allergy encountered clinically. This generalization applies to milk allergy in spite of the large number of studies reporting the immune responses to cow's milk proteins, both in healthy subjects and in milk-sensitive patients.

IMMUNE RESPONSES TO COW'S MILK PROTEINS IN HEALTHY PERSONS

Circulating antibodies against cow's milk proteins have been detected in healthy people by various immunologic techniques. Many authors have pointed out that several factors influence the immune response to cow's milk proteins. As early as 1923, precipitating antibodies against cow's milk were demonstrated in many children fed on cow's milk.[1] Gunther et al.,[2] using the tanned erythrocyte hemagglutination technique, found antibodies to cow's milk proteins in only one-half of sera from normal adults and in less than one-half of cord blood samples. The antibody titers were generally low in cord sera and in adult sera. Of infants between 7 and 97 weeks of age, however, 98 percent showed circulating antibodies to cows milk proteins, with the highest titers at ages 3 to 6 months. By means of the Farr technique of precipitating antibody and its bound radio-labeled antigen with ammonium sulfate, Rothberg and Farr[3] measured antibodies to bovine serum albumin and alpha-lactalbumin in well individuals. They noted that such antibodies were more frequent among children (41 to 74 percent) than among young adults (13 to 30 percent) or adults over 40 years (5 to 10 percent). In normal newborn infants, circulating antibodies to cow's milk proteins were usually absent or present in low titers. With the feeding of cow's milk, the antibody titer gradually rose and sometimes reached detectable levels within a few days. A similar pattern was observed by Kletter et al.[4] using the hemagglutination and radioimmunodiffusion techniques. In instances where circulating antibodies to cow's milk proteins were detected at birth, the antibodies were of the IgG class and the titers were comparable to those in the mother's circulation. With the feeding of pasteurized cow's milk, hemagglutinating antibodies were noted to rise during the first month, reaching a peak at about 3 months of age and then slowly declining (Fig. 4-1). Antibodies of the IgG class detected by radioimmunodiffusion followed a similar pattern, whereas IgA antibodies developed more slowly and peaked at 7 months of age. On the other hand, IgM antibodies were produced in the least quantity and did not show significant changes through the 12-month period of study. These findings support the earlier observations of Lippard et al.[5] using the complement fixation test.

Infants who were initially breast-fed for some time and later were given cow's milk showed slower and lesser production of hemagglutinating IgG and IgA antibodies to cow's milk proteins than infants fed cow's milk from birth, although the serum levels of total IgG, IgA, and IgM were similar in the two groups.[2,6,7]

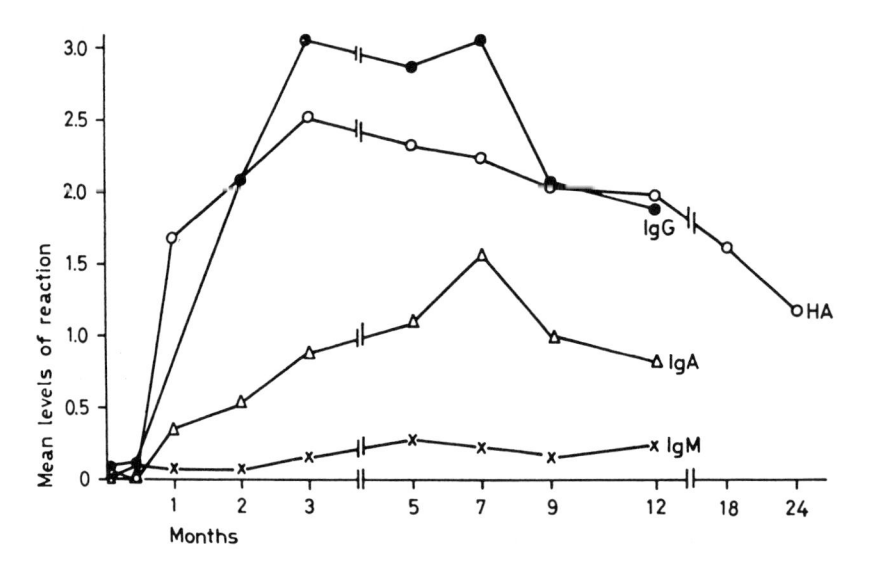

Fig. 4-1. Production of different types of antibodies to milk proteins in normal infants fed pasteurized cow's milk (HA-hemagglutination mean tube number; IgG, IgA, and IgM-radioimmunodiffusion mean reaction). From Kletter B, Gery I, Freier S, Davies AM: Immune responses of normal infants to cow's milk. I. Antibody type and kinetics of production. Int Arch Allergy Appl Immunol 40:656–666, 1971; S Karger AG, Basel. Reproduced with permission.

Using the enzyme-linked immunosorbent assay (ELISA), Hanson et al.[8] could demonstrate circulating antibodies to cow's milk proteins of the IgG, IgA, and IgM classes in normal infants who had mixed feeding—sometimes breast milk and sometimes cow's milk formula. Interestingly, IgG antibody titers were higher in infants who were weaned off the breast after a short period than in those who received mixed feeding for longer durations.

In newborn infants, agglutinating antibodies against cow's milk casein were noted to belong to the IgG class only, which suggested transfer across the placenta from the maternal circulation. Fällström et al.[9] reported that infants with clinical reactions to cow's milk as a group had higher levels of IgE and IgG antibodies than other patients or controls, whereas patients with gluten-induced enteropathy had increased levels of IgG and IgA antibodies. They found that with the ELISA method combined patterns of specific antibodies of different immunoglobulin classes often permitted discrimination of late clinically reacting individuals from controls.

In older infants fed cow's milk, both IgA and IgM antibodies were commonly found along with IgG antibodies, the latter usually present in the highest titer.[10] Using the radioimmunodiffusion technique, Rothberg[11] noted that premature infants fed bovine serum albumin were capable of producing antibovine serum albumin of both the IgG and IgM classes. The capacity to produce specific antibodies to bovine serum albumin was evident by the 35th week of gestation.[12]

Reagins (IgE antibodies) to cow's milk proteins in normal persons have been less frequently reported than antibodies of other immunoglobulin classes. In a group of 23 infants under one year of age who had been fed cow's milk, the radioimmunodiffusion technique failed to reveal any circulating IgE antibodies against beta-lactoglobulin, alpha-lactalbumin, or bovine gammaglobulin.[13,14] Parish,[15] however, using the techniques of passive cutaneous anaphylaxis in monkey, in vitro histamine release from passively sensitized human lung, radio-immunodiffusion and degranulation of passively sensitized monkey basophils, could detect antibeta-lactoglobulin reagins in a few normal adults. We have had considerable experience in studying antibodies to specific food proteins by the radioallergosorbent test (RAST), and we find that low levels of IgE antibodies to various food antigens, including cow's milk protein, are not uncommon in healthy subjects. Others have reported that low titers of IgE antibodies may be detected in more than one-half of normal infants. These usually decrease or disappear as children grow older.[16] By means of sensitive radioimmunoassays, IgD and IgG4 antibodies to many specific milk proteins can now be measured, whereas their presence was not detected by the methods available a decade ago. The time is now ripe for a gradual, more precise delineation of the specific roles of antibodies of individual immunoglobulin classes and subclasses in human health and disease.

Based on the studies outlined above, as well as on those by Matsumura et al.,[17] Dees,[18] May et al.,[19] and others, the presence of antibodies to cow's milk proteins in infants fed cow's milk can be a normal physiologic phenomenon. The form and degree of immunologic response to cow's milk proteins, however, depend on several factors, including:

1. Age of the infant at the time of introducing cow's milk in the diet. (The reaction is probably related to the maturity of the gastrointestinal tract and of the immune system, as will be discussed later in more detail.)
2. Mode of feeding, i.e., whether the feeding of cow's milk was preceded by or associated with breast-feeding.
3. Antigen load, i.e., quantity of cow's milk ingested.
4. Milk preparation consumed and the degree of denaturation of its proteins.
5. Individual variation with respect to the immune response, which is partly under genetic control.

It has been frequently noted, in outbred animals of a given species, and which have been immunized with the same antigen by the same technique, that some produce antibodies in higher quantities or of greater avidity than others, whereas less variation is noted in inbred strains. In man, serial serum samples obtained from the same person who is frequently exposed to a food antigen show greater consistency in the antibody response than is observed in sera from different persons similarly exposed to the same antigen.

IMMUNE RESPONSES TO COW'S MILK PROTEINS IN MILK-SENSITIVE PATIENTS

Since production of antibodies to cow's milk proteins is a common phenomenon in healthy persons, one immediately asks the question does the immune response to cow's milk proteins in milk-sensitive subjects differ from that in a control population. The answer appears to be yes, but only under certain circumstances. A few kinds of milk-sensitive patients tend to have antibodies to cow's milk proteins in higher titers than healthy persons, but the relationship is not sufficiently consistent to form the basis for a diagnostic test and the present time. In individual cases, one cannot expect a direct relationship between antibody titers and symptoms. There is probably greater discriminatory efficiency when several classes of antibody are evaluated, as suggested by Fällström et al.[9] This approach, however, is yet in its beginning stages and its exploitation will depend on continued improvements in laboratory tests.

Hypersensitivity reactions to cow's milk proteins, as well as to other foods, obviously involve more than one immunologic mechanism. Some types of hypersensitivity reaction are associated with the production of certain predominant antibodies such as IgE antibodies. In other instances, the immune response may be largely of the cell-mediated rather than of the humoral type.

When a microslide technique of double diffusion in agar is used, multiple precipitin lines (often five or more) are formed by the reaction between cow's milk and the sera of many patients with a milk-induced syndrome that includes chronic upper and lower respiratory tract disease and sometimes pulmonary hemosiderosis.[20-22] A somewhat similar group of patients was studied by Holland et al.,[23] who reported that hepatomegaly could accompany respiratory symptoms and precipitins to milk proteins. In a group of infants preponderantly with gastrointestinal cow's milk allergy, high hemagglutinating and precipitating antibodies were detected in one-half.[24]

Sera of patients with gastrointestinal milk allergy frequently contain antimilk precipitins rather than antimilk reagins.[15-25] Collins-Williams and Salama[26] noted an increased frequency of positive passive cutaneous anaphylaxis and precipitin tests in their group of milk-sensitive patients, whereas results from hemagglutinating tests did not differ from those of tests done on controls.

Milk precipitins or hemagglutinins are rarely elevated in association with classic atopic symptoms caused by the ingestion of cow's milk.[27-29] The antibodies usually encountered in atopic diseases, including atopic food allergy, are of the IgE class. The most helpful tests to identify and roughly measure IgE reagins are scratch and prick skin tests, RAST, leukocyte histamine release, radioimmunodiffusion, and crossed radioimmunoelectrophoresis (CRIE).

Involvement of complement in some instances of cow's milk allergy has been suggested by the observation of a fall in β1c level together with the detection of altered complement component in some milk-sensitive patients after oral milk challenge.[30, 31] Possibly some food protein molecules can activate complement directly.[32]

In recent years, several studies have shown that cell-mediated immunity may play an important role in certain manifestations of cow's milk allergy. Scheinmann et al.[33] carried out in vitro lymphoblast transformation on 45 patients with gastrointestinal milk intolerance. Positive results were obtained in 17 patients (38 percent): 8 with beta-lactoglobulin; 7 with alpha-lactalbumin; and 2 with both. In addition to lymphoblast transformation, lymphokine production has been assayed with some success.[34-37a] Accuracy in assessing lymphokine production will be enhanced when radioimmunoassays or specific chemical tests replace the biologic assays now used.

In addition to the above-mentioned immune responses, cow's milk allergy may involve IgG short-term sensitizing antibody, antigen-antibody complex formation and deposition, release of chemical mediators and modulators such as prostaglandins, kallikrein, Hageman factor, and possibly other systems.[32, 38, 39]

INTRAUTERINE SENSITIZATION

In 1928, Ratner[40] demonstrated intrauterine sensitization to cow's milk proteins in Guinea pigs, and warned that an analogous process might occur in man. Indeed, this seems to be the case in the occasional instance in which an infant develops an unequivoal allergic reaction after the first exposure to a food antigen, often cow's milk. If the validity of maternofetal transfer of food antigens is assumed, an immune response in the fetus would not be too surprising, since the capacity to synthesize immunoglobulins occurs as early as 8 to 12 weeks of gestation.[41-43] Actually, premature infants of 35 weeks of gestation were found to be capable of producing specific antibodies to cow's milk proteins.[11, 12] Acute hypersensitivity reactions occasionally occur in breast-fed infants after the first cow's milk meal.[9] Prenatal sensitization was suggested in five infants who developed exzema on the first postnatal exposure to cow's milk (three infants) and to soybean formula (two infants); hemagglutinating antibody titers against lactalbumin in the former infants and against soybean in the latter infants were elevated in the amniotic fluid.[44] We, as well as others,[45] have seen breast-fed neonates who had allergy symptoms to foods that were often ingested by the mother in excessive quantities during pregnancy. In one reported instance, the result of the RAST on the cord serum was positive for cow's milk.[46] We have found several cord sera which contained reagins to cow's milk protein.

ROLE OF GASTROINTESTINAL TRACT

The fact that hypersensitivity to cow's milk and to foods in general is much more common among infants than among older children or adults has led to a general belief that physiologic immaturity of the gastrointestinal tract might be a major factor. This point of view has been supported by the clinical observation that most young infants with food allergy are able to tolerate the offending food by the age of 1 or 2 years. Additional support comes from the observation that circulating hemagglutinating and precipitating antibodies against cow's milk proteins are present in many healthy infants, sometimes in high titer, but in a much smaller percentage of healthy adults. Perhaps the permeability of the mucosa of the gastrointestinal tract to intact macromolecules is more in infants than in adults. Infants fed cow's milk or soy protein formula from birth have been found to show considerably higher serum levels of agglutinins to milk or to soy proteins than those fed such proteins only after 3 months of age.[47] Antigenic competition may also be a factor. Thus, when a large proportion of the foreign antigen load to which a newborn infant is initially exposed consists of cow's milk proteins, a sizable proportion of the humoral immune response capability may be directed toward the cow's milk proteins. At a later age, after exposure to many other antigens and while being exposed to a larger number of antigens than in the newborn period, the proportion of the humoral immune response capability that can be directed toward cow's milk proteins may be smaller. Other factors may also be considered.

As early as 1904, the absorption of undigested egg protein was demonstrat-

Pathogenesis

ed by precipitin tests on sera of two debilitated infants.[48] A similar observation was noted by Modigliani and Benini in 1915[49] with respect to absorption of unaltered cow's milk casein. Schloss and Worthen,[50] using precipitin and guinea pig anaphylactic tests, noted that in infants with gastrointestinal disorders, cow's milk or egg protein may be absorbed in an undigested state, remain briefly in the circulation, and also be excreted in the urine for a few hours. By means of the passive transfer test, Walzer[51] and Wilson and Walzer[52] noted that the absorption of intact protein molecules is a common phenomenon in normal children. The intestinal permeability to undigested protein may be enhanced in the presence of diarrhea and decrease again on recovery.[53] Gamo et al.[54] detected bovine casein antigen in human serum by its reaction with ^{131}I-labeled rabbit anticasein gamma globulin. They noted that high "casein" levels were more common in sera of normal bottle-fed infants than in sera of adults, and that the levels were relatively independent of milk intake.

When the intestinal absorption of immunologically intact food proteins was studied, interesting information was obtained by means of three techniques:[55]

1. Precipitin tests detected circulating food antigens. In the sera of a few patients the simultaneous presence of a milk protein and antibodies to other milk proteins has been repeatedly demonstrated. Also, precipitins formed between two sera from different patients in Ouchterlony studies in some instances were shown to be a result of a circulating food antigen in one serum and antibodies specific to the same antigen in the other serum.
2. Production of specific antibodies to a food protein could occasionally be induced in rabbits injected with human sera. Antigens of cow's milk, wheat, or egg in sera of human subjects may occasionally be detected in this manner.
3. When a human serum containing skin-fixing antibodies to wheat gliadin was injected intradermally into normal human subjects, a positive reaction at the injection site was obtained after oral ingestion of gliadin. Furthermore, oral doses per kilogram of body weight of gliadin required to induce a positive reaction in newborn infants was about one-tenth that required in older children. That difference may reflect a greater permeability of the intestinal mucosa in younger infants[55-58] than in adults.[54,59] Intestinal permeability seems to be especially increased in prematurely born infants.[11,12] Recent studies have suggested an important role of feeding breast milk in accelerating intestinal maturation in the newborn. Adding cell-free human milk supernatant to intestinal lymphoid cells obtained from young children resulted in a significant enhancement of IgA production.[60] In another study, the intestinal permeability to macromolecules in newborn rabbits was less in maternally-fed than in formula-fed animals.[61]

Many studies[62-68] have shown that the mature gastrointestinal tract is equipped with defense mechanisms to hinder the penetration of antigenic material. The mucosal barrier, however, is by no means a complete one, particularly in early infancy.

The general mechanism of transport of antigens across the intestinal mucosa probably involves several steps (Fig. 4-2). After the adsorption of macromolecules onto the microvillus membrane, the membrane is locally invaginated (endocytosis), and the macromolecules become enclosed in small vacuoles by means of an energy-dependent movement. Such vacuoles migrate from the luminal surface of the cell toward the center of the cell and coalesce, forming larger vacuoles (phagosomes). The latter merge with the intracellular lysosomes to form larger vacuoles (phagolysosomes), in which intracellular digestion of the particulate material occurs. Particles that remain undigested migrate within small vacuoles toward the basal surface of the cell to be released from the vacuoles (exocytosis) and become deposited in the interstitial space. When increased quantities of macromolecules traverse the intestinal epithelial cell, they have a higher chance of absorption into the lymphatics and of entering the systemic circulation. Fac-

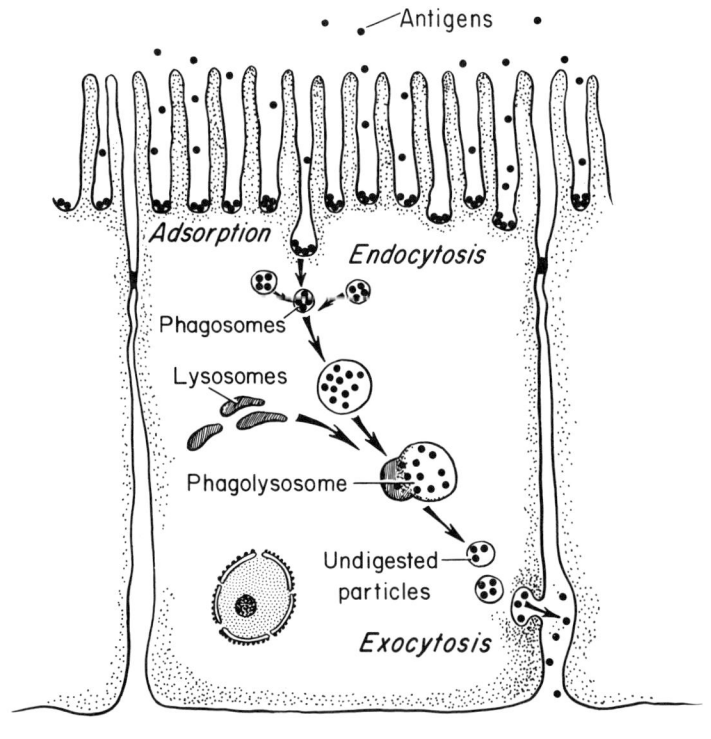

Fig. 4-2. General mechanism for the uptake and transport of antigens by the intestinal epithelial cell. From Walker WA, Isselbacher KJ: Uptake and transport of macromolecules by the intestine: Possible role in clinical disorders. Gastroenterology 67:531–550, 1974. Reproduced with permission.

tors that may enhance excessive absorption of macromolecules include incomplete intraluminal digestion, injured intestinal mucosa, and reduced secretory IgA.[70] Experimental studies on rats showed that the absorption of intact antigenic protein is much greater from the small intestine than from the colon.[67] Immunologically, the intestinal wall contains abundant lymphoid tissue, mainly aggregrated in Peyer's patches as well as diffusely spread throughout in the lamina propria. Plasma cells in the lamina propria are capable of producing all classes or immunoglobulins, but especially IgA.[62, 63, 66]

The immune system probably plays a role locally in hindering the absorption of macromolecules, and systemically in neutralizing the antigen molecules that gain access to the circulation. After antigen ingestion, specific antibodies may be detected in the intestinal secretions or the stools (coproantibodies).[71-74]

In a study of infants with gastrointestinal milk allergy, Kletter et al.[75] using a radioimmunoelectrophoretic technique, found that antibodies to cow's milk proteins in the stools belong mainly to the IgA class, with smaller amounts in the IgG class. Circulating antibodies, on the other hand, showed a reverse preponderance. Also, there was little correlation between the levels of coproantibodies and of serum antibodies, suggesting that the local intestinal immune response is independent of the systemic response. The concept is substantiated by the findings of Ogra and Karzon[73] on children with double-barrel surgical colostomy. Instillation of live poliovirus vaccine in the distal segment was followed by the appearance in the immunized segment of antibodies strictly of the IgA class and in much higher titers than in the proximal segment of the colon. On the other hand, serum antibodies were mainly of the IgG class, whereas IgA antibodies were late in appearance and in much lower titers than IgG antibodies. Some studies also suggest that sensitized lymphocytes in the lamina propria of the small intestine may enter the circulation, then "home" to exocrine glands, including active mammary glands, where they continue to generate antibodies (mainly of the IgA class) against the originally ingested antigen[76-79a] (Fig. 4-3).

ROLE OF SECRETORY IgA

In contrast to the circulation and peripheral lymphoid tissue where IgG is the preponderant immunoglobulin, in the gastrointestinal tract the principal immunoglobulin is IgA.[63, 80-83] By means of immunofluorescent techniques, the plasma cells in the lamina propria of the intestine have been shown to be primarily IgA-producing cells.[84, 85] IgA produced by such cells is a dimer joined together by a polypeptide chain called joining "J" chain (molecular weight 15,000 daltons). From the lamina propria, IgA reaches the epithelial surface of the mucosa by an intracellular transport process, during which it acquires a glycoprotein moiety designated the "secretory piece".[86, 87] In addition to its possible role in the intracellular transport of IgA,[88] the secretory piece renders IgA resistant to

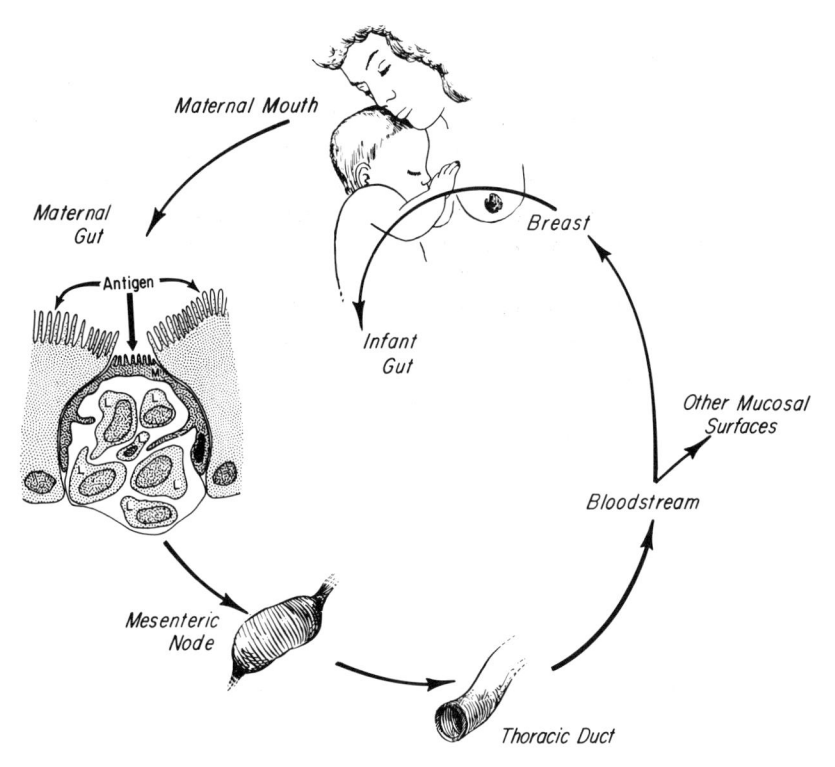

Fig. 4-3. The enteromammary circulation of lymphocytes. The antigen that enters the mother's gut is brought into proximity to lymphoid cells (L) by special transport cells (M). The lymphoid cells become committed to specific IgA antibody production, and they then migrate via the lymphatics to the mesenteric nodes and thoracic duct into the systemic circulation. During periods of proper hormonal stimulation, these cells populate the mammary gland and produce SIgA against the original antigen ingested by the mother. From Kleinman RE, Walker WA: The enteromammary immune system: An important new concept in breast milk host defense. Dig Dis Sci 24:876–882, 1979. Reproduced with permission.

proteolytic enzymes and pH changes.[89,90] In its final form, secretory IgA is a dimer with a sedimentation coefficient of 11S and molecular weight of 390,000 daltons, whereas serum IgA is largely a 7S monomer with molecular weight of 170,000 daltons, and is more easily destroyed by proteolytic enzymes.

At the mucosal surface, SIgA antibodies tend to remain within the mucus coat because of interaction with cystine residues contained in mucin.[91] SIgA antibodies may function through a process of immune exclusion, in which the antibodies interact with antigens and prevent their adherence to or uptake by the intestinal epithelial cells.[66]

Patients with selective IgA deficiency frequently have gastrointestinal disorders.[92,93] The lamina propria shows a considerable increase in the number of IgM-producing cells, and the intestinal secretion contains an increased quantity of IgM.[94] Although the capacity to synthesize IgA and other immunoglobulins develops in the fetus as early as 8 to 12 weeks of gestation,[41,43] under normal circumstances both serum and secretory IgA are very low or even absent in the newborn infant.[95,96] At birth, the lamina propria is usually devoid of IgA-producing plasma cells, and it may take several weeks for an antigen exposure to induce detectable levels of intestinal secretory IgA antibodies.[97] Transient IgA deficiency at 3 months of age has been noted by Taylor et al.[98] in infants of atopic parents, and the IgA levels were especially low for those who subsequently showed atopic manifestations during the first year of life. Perhaps, the local intestinal immune system in the newborn may be considered immature and incapable of handling a high antigen load.[70,99,100] In the potentially allergic infant, an increased absorption of intact antigens may sensitize the infant, and then with subsequent reexposure even to a small quantity of antigen, allergy symptoms may occur. Deficiency of IgA was present in an unusually high incidence in atopic children, especially during infancy.[101] In one series of children with cow's milk protein intolerance, a partial IgA deficiency was noted in 40 percent.[102] Development of food allergy may also be enhanced during transient hypogammaglobulinemia of infancy.[103]

A strong correlation was noted between selective IgA deficiency and the presence of circulating precipitins or hemagglutinins against cow's milk proteins.[104] Milk precipitins were detected in 40 to 75 percent of patients with selective IgA deficiency,[104-107] and the precipitins were commonly directed to bovine IgM. The high incidence of these precipitins in patients with selective IgA deficiency is of particular importance, since they may conceal the absence of IgA in the serum sample by formation of antiantiserum precipitin rings in radial immunodiffusion.[105] Furthermore, in patients with selective IgA deficiency, the presence of precipitating antibodies to cow's milk proteins or to bovine serum proteins has been associated with detectable circulating immune complexes in quantities correlating with the precipitin titers.[106] After an IgA-deficient patient had ingested 100 ml of cow's milk, sequential serum samples showed the presence of casein in the circulation at 1 hour and the appearance of increasing amounts of immune complexes for 2 hours.[106] In that particular patient, interestingly enough, free casein was detected in the circulation only during the interval in which immune complexes were not detected.

IMMUNOLOGIC MECHANISMS

The existence of more than one immunologic mechanism in milk allergy was suggested as early as 1948, when Vendel[108] recognized immediate and delayed onset reactions in patients with cow's milk idiosyncrasy. Our present understanding of the immune mechanisms underlying food allergy is somewhat improved over that of a few years ago, but much remains to be learned. Part of the problem is related to the fact that circulating antibodies against cow's milk proteins are frequently detected in apparently healthy persons, whereas they are not demonstrable in some patients with symptoms attributable to milk ingestion. That fact should not be surprising, since antibodies in proper amounts and in a well-balanced immune system are protective and they assist in maintaining health. We now suspect that immune mechanisms are out of balance or improperly "tuned" in most cases of food allergy and other kinds of hypersensitivity. Evidence is convincing that more than one type of immunologic mechanism is operative in most immune reponses, including those resulting in allergic symptoms.

Currently the most widely used classification of allergic mechanisms is that of Gell and Coombs,[109] who propose four basic types:

1. *Type I, anaphylactic or immediate hypersensitivity.* This type of response is initiated by a reaction between the allergen or antigen and its specific IgE (or short-term IgG) antibody on the surface of mast cells, resulting in the release of chemical mediators that increase local blood flow, vascular permeability, and attract a variety of mobile cells into the site of local reaction.
2. *Type II, cytotoxic or cytolytic.* In this reaction antibody (usually of the IgG or IgM class) reacts with an antigenic component of a cell. The antigen may be part of the cell structure or an exogenous antigen or hapten adsorbed to the cell surface. Complement fixation and activation usually participate in producing cytolysis and tissue damage.
3. *Type III, Arthus-like or immune-complex.* The antigen combines with specific antibody (IgG or IgM), generally in the presence of antigen excess, with subsequent complement fixation and the formation of circulating immune complexes. The latter cause vasculitis, local inflammatory responses, and tissue damage. Complement-derived chemotactic factors attract polymorphonuclear leukocytes to the reaction site, some of which become destroyed and release proteolytic enzymes that cause tissue damage as well.
4. *Type IV, delayed hypersensitivity or cell-mediated reaction.* Sensitized T-lymphocytes migrate to the site where antigen is present and react with the target cell or microorganism harboring the antigen. At the same time, such T-cells release a variety of reactive substances called lymphokines, which facilitate the immune responses, and often participate in tissue damage.

At least three of these types of reactions (I, III, IV), and probably all four can be involved in varying degrees in milk allergy.

Anaphylactic Reactions

Anaphylactic reactions are primarily IgE-mediated but in a few instances other mechanisms must play an important role, since no evidence for IgE antibodies can be found. The reaction occurs within minutes to a few hours after

Pathogenesis 35

exposure to the allergens, it usually improves within hours, and it disappears within 24 to 48 hours after avoidance of the allergen. The onset of symptoms may be more rapid when the released chemical mediator is largely histamine rather than SRS-A or kinins.[110] The presenting symptoms vary considerably, from systemic anaphylaxis to wheezing, vomiting, diarrhea, abdominal pain, urticaria, angioedema, eczema, or rhinitis. They are often provoked by small quantities of allergen, which may result in severe symptoms in highly sensitive subjects. Severe reactions are rare in milk allergy, but the physician should be aware of their possible occurrence and be prepared for prompt management. The frequency of this type of reaction in milk allergy varies from one series to another and is probably responsible for about one-fourth to one-third of reactions to milk. A rise in the serum IgE level and an increase in the eosinophils in the circulation or in the local secretion are often present.

Specific tests that may be helpful in detecting reagins to milk, and thus support the likelihood that immediate-type immune response is involved, include the following:

1. Skin-testing. Testing the skin remains the simplest and the most frequently used technique in identifying immediate-type hypersensitivity.
2. Radioallergosorbent test (RAST)[111-113].
3. Crossed radioimmunoelectrophoresis in gel. Specific milk proteins are electrophoresed and precipitated with rabbit antisera, then the patient's serum is applied to the precipitate, and finally the serum IgE antibody is detected by applying radio-labeled anti-IgE.[25]
4. Passive cutaneous anaphylaxis in monkey using the patient's serum.[114]
5. Prausnitz-Küstner reaction.[100] This technique is seldom used because of the risk of hepatitis.
6. Leukocyte histamine release.[34, 115, 116]
7. Histamine release from human lung tissue passively sensitized in vitro.[117]
8. Degranulation of passively sensitized monkey basophils.[15]
9. Radioimmunodiffusion.[13, 118]
10. Immunofluorescence studies on small-bowel biopsy[112, 119]

Most of these tests will be discussed in greater detail in Chapter 6 (Diagnosis).

Immune Complex Reactions

Immune complex reactions usually involve relatively large quantities of antigen that combine with specific antibodies to form immune complexes. These reactions are most likely to result in tissue damage when there is slight to moderate antigen excess, but in at least one model the greatest damage was induced by complexes at antigen-antibody equivalence.[120] Complement fixed to the antigen-antibody complexes may result in a fall in the level of serum complement.[30] The antibodies involved in these reactions are thought to be largely of the IgG (IgG1, IgG2, and IgG3) or IgM classes, which are capable of fixing complement through the classic pathway. Stafford et al.[121] noted in milk-induced pulmonary hemosiderosis an association between serum milk precipitins and the presence of high concentrations of milk antibodies of the IgG and IgA but not of the IgM or IgE classes. In some instances, however, an associated IgE-mediated reaction may enhance the deposition of immune complexes.[122] Microprecipitates formed by the complexes may initiate an acute inflammatory reaction in the endothelium of small blood vessels and leads to vasculitis.

The symptoms usually appear 6 to 12 hours or a few days after exposure to the allergen and may last for several days to a few weeks. Because of the delayed onset, a cause-effect relationship between the food ingested and appearance of symptoms may not be evident. The symptoms may not disappear until the allergen has been eliminated for a few days or weeks.

This type of reaction may be responsible for as many as one-half of milk hypersensitivity manifestations, although no data are available on its frequency. It is possibly involved in milk-induced gross intestinal bleeding in infants,[123] occult intestinal bleeding,[124] gastroenteropathy,[125] pulmonary hemosiderosis,[21,22,121] and certain cases of renal disease.[126,127] Findings that may indicate this type of reaction include high titers of precipitins or hemagglutinins, complement-fixing antibodies, lowered serum complement components, and detection of circulating immune complexes.

In a patient with circulating immune complexes consisting of bovine gamma globulin and antibovine gamma globulin, immunofluorescence studies on a renal biopsy revealed patchy granular glomerular deposits with antibovine gamma globulin.[128] In addition to circulating immune complexes, antibodies to a microsomal ubiquitous tissue antigen were demonstrated in the serum of a patient with classic milk-induced gastroenteropathy.[129]

Cell-mediated Reactions

Delayed-type hypersensitivity reactions are lymphocyte-mediated, and need not involve the humoral immune system. Reactions generally occur 24 to 72 hours after exposure to the allergen and may last for several days after a single exposure. The reaction results in a subacute inflammatory response involving cell damage and tissue destruction that may become chronic with continued exposure to the antigen.

The frequency of this type of reaction in milk allergy is not known, mainly because of the lack of a reliable practical diagnostic test. It is probably involved in several manifestations of milk allergy, including certain types of gastroenteropathy and dermatitis from direct contact with milk. Skin-testing may be of help if there is a positive response after 24 to 48 hours. In vitro lymphoblast transformation of the patient's lymphocytes may occur in the presence of the offending protein antigen, and this may be accompanied by antigen-induced lymphokine production.

Scheinmann et al.[33] noted in vitro milk-induced lymphoblast transformation of peripheral blood lymphocytes in 17 out of 45 patients (38 percent) with gastrointestinal cow's milk intolerance. The same authors also noted that the children with the most severe symptoms had the highest incidence of lymphoblast transformation (46 percent). Other investigators[34-36] also noted blast transformation and release of lymphokines when lymphocytes of patients with delayed hypersensitivity to milk were incubated with cow's milk protein antigens. In some instances, lymphocytes taken from the patients ingesting milk or after a milk challenge show in vitro proliferation without the addition of antigen, suggesting that the cells may be stimulated by the antigen in vivo. Such stimulation may persist for several days or weeks after ingesting the food allergen.[130]

A comparison of the three major immune mechanisms that have been recognized in milk allergy is summarized in Table 4-1.

In many milk-sensitive patients, routine immunologic studies may fail to demonstrate unusual circulating antibodies to cow's milk proteins. Because of this important fact, some workers have investigated the possibility that new allergens form as a result of protein digestion in the gastrointestinal tract. In fact, that theory was suggested by Cooke in 1942[131] as a explanation of the negative results of skin-testing to known food allergens. In vitro pepsin digestion of bovine serum albumin, alpha-lactalbumin, beta-lactoglobulin, and casein resulted in the production of new antigens, some of which formed precipitates with rabbit antisera whereas others did not. Eight new antigens could be generated by successive pepsin hydrolysis of beta-lactoglobulin.[132] Recently Haddad et al.[133] reported that some children with milk hypersensitivity in whom IgE antibodies determined by RAST to whole cow's milk or to individual cow's milk protein fractions were negative, had positive responses when discs coated with pepsin digests or pepsin-trypsin digests of cow's milk protein were used. Nevertheless, most antigens recognized in milk protein digests by serum antibodies of patients are also present on the native proteins where they are similarly reactive with the patient's antibodies. Up to the present time no critical studies have shown that a hypersensitivity response was produced in man solely by new antigens produced in the gastrointestinal tract.

As improved laboratory techniques are exploited in the study of hypersensitivity to foods, many subtle variations and combinations of immune responses will probably be found.

Table 4-1
Presumed Mechanisms in Cow's Milk Allergy

Immunologic Reaction	Immediate Hypersensitivity	Immune Complex	Delayed Hypersensitivity
Gell and Coombs classification	Type I	Type III	Type IV
Mediated by	IgE or short-term IgG	Immune complexes	T lymphocytes
Onset of symptoms	Minutes to a few hours	4 to 12 hours	24 to 72 hours
Usual duration	Minutes to a few hours	Few hours to a few days	Several days
Predominates in	Anaphylaxis	GI bleeding	Contact dermatitis
	Urticaria, angioedema	Protein-losing enteropathy	Tension-fatigue syndrome
	Facilitating vasculitis	Malabsorption	
	Atopic dermatitis	Pulmonary disease	
	Rhinitis, asthma	Vasculitis, purpura	
	Vomiting, diarrhea		
Usually increased	Eosinophils	Precipitins	Lymphoblast transformation
	Leukocyte histamine release	Hemagglutinins	Lymphokine production
	Total IgE	Complement activation	
	IgE antibody		
Maximal skin response	Erythema and wheal in 10 to 20 min	Induration or nonpitting edema in 4 to 8 hr	Induration in 24 to 48 hr

REFERENCES

1. Anderson AF, Schloss DM: Allergy to cow's milk in infants with nutritional disorders: A preliminary report. Am J Dis Child 26:451–474, 1923
2. Gunther M, Aschaffenburg R, Matthews RH, et al.: The level of antibodies to the proteins of cow's milk in the serum of normal human infants. Immunology 3:296–306, 1960
3. Rothberg RM, Farr RS: Anti-bovine serum albumin and anti-alpha lactalbumin in the serum of children and adults. Pediatrics 35:571–588, 1965
4. Kletter B, Gery I, Freier S, et al.: Immune responses of normal infants to cow's milk. I. Antibody type and kinetics of production. Int Arch Allergy Appl Immunol 40:656–666, 1971
5. Lippard VW, Schloss OM, Johnson PA: Immune reactions induced in infants by intestinal absorption of incompletely digested cow's milk proteins. Am J Dis Child 51:562–574, 1936
6. Gunther M, Cheek E, Matthews RH, et al.: Immune responses in infants to cow's milk proteins taken by mouth. Int Arch Allergy 21:257–278, 1962
7. Kletter B, Gery I, Freier S, et al.: Immune responses of normal infants to cow's milk. II. Decreased immune reactions in initially breast-fed infants. Int Arch Allergy Appl Immunol 40:667–674, 1971
8. Hanson LÅ, Ahlstedt S, Carlsson B, et al.: Secretory IgA antibodies against cow's milk proteins in human milk and their possible effect in mixed feeding. Int Arch Allergy Appl Immunol 54:457–462, 1977
9. Fällström ŠP, Ahlstedt S, Hanson LÅ: Specific antibodies in infants with gastrointestinal intolerance to cow's milk protein. Int Arch Allergy Appl Immunol 56:97–105, 1978
10. Hunter A, Feinstein A, Coombs RRA: Immunoglobulin class of antibodies to cow's milk casein in infant sera and evidence for low molecular weight IgM antibodies. Immunology 15:381–388, 1968
11. Rothberg RM: Immunoglobulin and specific antibody synthesis during the first weeks of life of premature infants. J Pediatr 75:391–399, 1969
12. Reiger CHL, Rothberg RM: Development of the capacity to produce specific antibody to an ingested food antigen in the premature infant. J Pediatr 87:515–518, 1975
13. Kletter B, Gery I, Frier S, et al.: Immunoglobulin E antibodies to milk proteins. Clin Allergy 1:249–255, 1971
14. Freier S, Kletter B: Clinical and immunological aspects of milk protein intolerance. Aust Paediatr J 8:140–146, 1972
15. Parish WE: Detection of reaginic and short-term sensitizing anaphylactic or anphylactoid antibodies to milk in sera of allergic and normal persons. Clin Allergy 1:369–380, 1971
16. Foucard T: A follow-up study of children with asthmatoid bronchitis. Acta Paediatr Scand 62:633–644, 1973
17. Matsumara T, Kuroume T, Mitonio A, et al.: Age differences of BDB hemagglutinating antibody titers against milk and egg allergens. Int Arch Allergy 30:341–350, 1966
18. Dees SC: Some unresolved problems in clinical allergy: Observations on milk and egg hemagglutinating antibody titers in allergic children. Pediatrics 50:420–428, 1972
19. May CD, Remigio L, Feldman J, et al.: A study of serum antibodies to isolated milk proteins and ovalbumin in infants and children. Clin Allergy 7:583–595, 1977
20. Heiner DC, Sears JW: Chronic respiratory disease associated with multiple circulating precipitins to cow's milk. Am J Dis Child 100:500–502, 1960
21. Heiner DC, Sears JW, Kniker WT: Multiple precipitins to cow's milk in chronic respiratory disease. Am J Dis Child 103:634–654, 1962
22. Lee SK, Kniker WT, Cook CD, Heiner DC: Cow's milk induced pulmonary disease in children, in Barness LA, et al. (eds): Advances in Pediatrics, vol 25. Chicago, Year Book, 1978, pp 39–57

23. Holland NH, Hong R, Davis NC, et al.: Significance of precipitating antibodies to milk proteins in the serum of infants and children. J Pediatr 61:181–195, 1962
24. Freier S, Kletter B, Gery I, et al.: Intolerance to milk protein. J Pediatr 75:623–631, 1969
25. Lowenstein H, Krasilnikoff PA, Bjerrrum OJ, et al.: Occurrence of specific precipitins against bovine whey proteins in serum from children with gastrointestinal disorders. Int Arch Allergy Appl Immunol 55:514–525, 1977
26. Collins-Williams C, Salama Y: A laboratory study in the diagnosis of milk allergy. Int Arch Allergy 27:110–128, 1965
27. Saperstein S, Anderson DW, Goldman AS, et al.: Immunological studies with sera from allergic and normal children. Pediatrics 32:580–587, 1963
28. Luz AQ, Todd RH: Antigenicity of heated milk proteins. Am J Dis Child 108:479–486, 1964
29. Bayless TM, Partin JS, Rosensweig NS: Absence of milk antibodies in milk intolerance in adults. JAMA 201:50, 1967
30. Matthews TS, Soothill JF: Complement activation after milk feeding in children with cow's milk allergy. Lancet 2:893–895, 1970
31. Iyngkaran N. Robinson MJ, Prathap K, et al.: Cow's milk protein sensitive enteropathy: Combined clinical and histological criteria for diagnosis. Arch Dis Child 53:20–26, 1978
32. Stroud RM: Complement activation and immune complexes in food allergy. Second International Food Allergy Symposium, Mexico City, October 17-20, 1978, pp 8–9
33. Scheinmann P, Gendrel D, Charles J, et al.: Value of lymphoblast transformation test in cow's milk protein intestinal intolerance. Clin Allergy 6:515–521, 1976
34. May CD, Alberto R: In-vitro responses of leucocytes to food proteins in allergic and normal children: Lymphocyte stimulation and histamine release. Clin Allergy 2:335–344, 1972
35. Baudon JJ, Fontaine JL, Mougenot JF, et al.: Digestive intolerance to cow's milk proteins in infants: Biological and histological study. Arch Fr Pediatr 32:787–801, 1975
36. Endré L, Osvath P: Antigen-induced lymphoblast transformation in the diagnosis of cow's milk allergic diseases in infancy and early childhood. Acta Allergol (Kbh) 30:34–42, 1975
37. Frick OL: Clinical evaluation and management of "delayed onset" food allergy. Second International Food Allergy Symposium, Mexico City, October 17–20, 1978, p 27
37a. Ashkenazi A, Levin S, Ider D, et al.: An immunological assay for sensitivity to cow's milk protein, X International Congress of Allergology. Jerusalem, November 4–11, 1979, p 9
38. Buisseret PD, Youlten LJF, Heinzelmann DI, et al.: Prostaglandin-synthesis inhibitors in prophylaxis of food intolerance. Lancet 1:906–908, 1978
39. Kaliner MA: Chemical mediators of mast cells. Second International Food Allergy Symposium, Mexico City, October 17–20, 1978, p 10
40. Ratner B: A possible causal-factor of food allergy in certain infants. Am J Dis Child 36:277–288, 1928
41. Gitlin D, Biasucci A: Development of $\gamma G, \gamma A, \gamma M$, β_{1c}/β_{1a}, $C'1$ esterase inhibitor, ceruloplasmin, transferrin, hemopexin, haptoglobin, fibrinogen, plasminogen, α_1-antitrypsin, orosomucoid, β-lipoprotein, α_2-macroglobulin and prealbumin in the human conceptus. J Clin Invest 48:1433–1446, 1969
42. Miller DL, Hirvonen T, Gitlin D: Synthesis of IgE by the human conceptus. J Allergy Clin Immunol 52:182–188, 1973
43. Singer AD, Hobel CJ, Heiner DC: Evidence for secretory IgA and IgE in utero. J Allergy Clin Immunol 53:94, 1974
44. Kuroume T, Oguri M, Matsumura T, et al.: Milk sensitivity and soybean sensitivity in the production of eczematous manifestations in breast-fed infants with particular reference to intrauterine sensitization. Ann Allergy 37:41–46, 1976
45. Gerrard JW: Allergy in breast fed babies to ingredients in breast milk. Ann Allergy 42:69–72, 1979

Pathogenesis

46. Frick OL, German DF, Mills J: Development of allergy in children. I. Association with virus infections. J Allergy Clin Immunol 63:228–241, 1979
47. Eastham EJ, Lichauco T, Grady MI, et al.: Antigenicity of infant formulas: Role of immature intestine on protein permeability. J Pediatr 93:561–564, 1978
48. Ganghofner, Langer J: Ueber die Resorption genuiner Eiweisskörper im Magendarmkonal neugeborener Tiere und Saüglinge. Munch Med Wochensehr li:1497–1502, 1904
49. Modigliani E, Benini R: Permeability of infant's intestine for casein of cow's milk. JAMA 64:476, 1915
50. Schloss OM, Worthen TW: The permeability of the gastro-enteric tract of infants to undigested protein. Am J Dis Child 11:342–360, 1916
51. Walzer M: A direct method of demonstrating the absorption of incompletely digested proteins in normal human beings. J Immunol 11:249–252, 1926
52. Wilson SJ, Walzer M: Absorption of undigested proteins in human beings. Am J Dis Child 50:49–54, 1935
53. Gruskay FL, Cooke RE: The gastrointestinal absorption of unaltered protein in normal infants, and in infants recovering from diarrhea. Pediatrics 16:763–769, 1955
54. Gamo I, Nishida M, Ikeda T, et al.: Studies on the antigenicity of cow's milk in infants. Med J Osaka Univ 18:397–415, 1968
55. Heiner DC: Intestinal absorption of immunologically intact food proteins. Soc Pediatr Res 63:744–747, 1963
56. Kane S: Nutritional management of allergic reactions to cow's milk. Am Practit 8:65–69, 1957
57. Sutton RE, Hamilton JR: Tolerance of young children with severe gastroenteritis to dietary lactose: A controlled study. Can Med Assoc J 99:980–982, 1968
58. Royer P: Breast feeding and biology of development, in Ghai OP (ed): New Developments in Pediatric Research, vol I. New Delhi, Interprint, 1977, p 32
59. Korenblat PE, Rothberg RM, Minden P, et al.: Immune responses of human adults after oral and parenteral exposure to bovine serum albumin. J Allergy 41:226–235, 1968
60. Gregoire RP, Halpin TC: Components of breast milk stimulate human intestinal lymphoid cell immunoglobuilin A biosynthesis. Pediatr Res 13:448, 1979
61. Udall JN, Pang K, Scrimshaw NS, et al.: The effect of early nutrition on intestinal maturation. Pediatr Res 13:409, 1979
62. Walker WA, Hong R: Immunology of the gastrointestinal tract: Part I. J Pediatr 83:517–530, 1973
63. Walker WA: Host defense mechanisms in the gastrointestinal tract. Pediatrics 57:901–916, 1976
64. Walker WA: Development of intestinal host defense mechanisms and the passive protective role of human milk. Mead Johnson Symp Perinat Dev Med 11:39–48, 1977
65. Parker CW: Immune responses to environmental antigens absorbed through the gastrointestinal tract. Fed Proc 36:1732–1735, 1977
66. Walker WA, Isselbacher KJ: Intestinal antibodies. N Engl J Med 297:767–773, 1977
67. Warshaw AL, Bellini CA, Walker WA: The intestinal mucosal barrier to intact antigenic protein: Difference between colon and small intestine. Am J Surg 133:55–58, 1978
68. Walker WA: Antigen handling by the gut. Arch Dis Child 53:527–531, 1978
69. Walker WA, Isselbacher, KJ: Uptake and transport of macromolecules by the intestine: Possible role in clinical disorders. Gastroenterology 67:531–550, 1974
70. Walker WA: Antigen absorption from the small intestine and gastrointestinal disease. Pediatr Clin North Am 22:731–746, 1975
71. Katz J, Spiro HM, Herskovic T: Milk precipitating substance in the stool in gastrointestinal milk sensitivity. N Engl J Med 278:1191–1194, 1968

72. Gryboski JD, Katz J, Reynolds D, et al.: Gluten intolerance following cow's milk sensitivity: Two cases with coproantibodies to milk and wheat proteins. Ann Allergy 26:33–39, 1968
73. Ogra PL, Karzon DT: Distribution of poliovirus antibody in serum, nasopharynx and alimentary tract following segmental immunization of lower alimentary tract with poliovaccine. J Immunol 102:1423–1430, 1969
74. Davis SD, Bierman CW, Pierson WE, et al.: Clinical nonspecificity of milk coproantibodies in diarrheal stools. N Engl J Med 282:612–613, 1970
75. Kletter B, Freier S, Davies AM, et al.: Coproantibodies to milk: Identification by radio immunoelectrophoresis. J Immunol 103:857–858, 1969
76. Gindrat JJ, Gothefors L, Hanson LÅ, et al.: Antibodies in human milk against *E. coli* of the serogroups most commonly found in neonatal infections. Acta Paediatr Scand 61:587–590, 1972
77. Montgomery PC, Cohn J, Lally ET: The indcution and characterization of secretory IgA antibody: The immunoglobulin A system. Adv Exp Med Biol 45:453–462, 1974
78. Goldblum RM, Ahlstredt S, Carlsson B, et al.: Antibody production by human colostrum cells. Pediatr Res 9:330, 1975
78a. Hanson LÅ, Ahlsted S, Carlsson B, et al.: Secretory IgA antibodies to enterobacterial virulence antigens: Their induction and possible relevance. Adv Exp Med Biol 107:165–176, 1978
79. Hanson LÅ, Ahlstedt S, Carlsson B, et al.: New knolwedge in human milk immunoglobulin. Acta Paediatr Scand 67:577–582, 1978
79a. Kleinman RE, Walker WA: The enteromammary immune system: An important new concept in breast milk host defense. Dig Dis Sci 24:876–882, 1979
80. Tomasi TB, Bienenstock J: Secretory immunoglobulin. Adv Immunol 9:1–96, 1968
81. Heremans JF: Immunoglobulin formation and function in different tissues. Curr Top Microbiol Immunol 45:131–203, 1968
82. Crabbé PA, Carbonara AO, Heremans JF: The normal human intestinal mucosa as a major source of plasma cells containing gamma A immunoglobulin. Lab Invest 14:235–248, 1965
83. Bienenstock J: The significance of secretory immunoglobulins. Can Med Assoc J 103:39–43, 1970
84. Crabbé PA, Heremans JF: The distribution of immunoglobulin containing cells along the human gastrointestinal tract. Gastroenterology 51:305–316, 1966
85. Van Furth R, Aiuti F: Immunoglobulin synthesis by tissues of the gastrointestinal and respiratory tracts. Protides Biol Fluids 16:479–484, 1968
86. Hanson LA, Johansson BG: Studies on secretory IgA, in Killander J (ed): Nobel Symposium on Gammaglobulins. Stockholm, Almqvist and Wiksell, 1967, pp 141–151
87. Halpern MS, Koshland ME: Novel subunit in secretory IgA. Nature (London) 228:1276–1278, 1970
88. Brown WR, Isobe Y, Nakane PK: Ultrastructural localization of IgA and secretory component (SC) in human intestinal mucosa by immunoperoxidase techniques. Gastroenterology 65:869, 1975
89. Tomasi TB, Tan EM, Solomon A, et al.: Characteristics of an immune system common to certain external secretions. J Exp Med 121:101–123, 1965
90. Lindh E: Increased resistance of immunoglobulin A dimers to proteolytic degradation after binding of secretory component. J Immunol 114:284–286, 1975
91. Bienenstock J: The local immune response. Am J Vet Res 36:488–491, 1975
92. Crabbé PA, Heremans JF: Selective IgA deficiency with steatorrhea: A new syndrome. Am J Med 42:319–325, 1967
93. Hong R, Ammann AJ: Selective absence of IgA. Am J Pathol 69:491–496, 1972

94. Douglas AP, Crabbé PA, Hobbs JR: Immunochemical studies of the serum, intestinal secretions and intestinal mucosa in patients with adult celiac disease and other forms of the celiac syndrome. Gastroenterology 59:414–425, 1970
95. South MA, Cooper MD, Wolheim FA, et al.: The IgA system. II. The clinical significance of IgA deficiency. Studies in patients with agammaglobulinemia and ataxia telangiectasia. Am J Med 44:168–178, 1968
96. Matthew DJ, Taylor B, Norman AP, et al.: Prevention of eczema. Lancet 1:321–324, 1977
97. Selner JC, Merrill DA, Claman HN: Salivary immunoglobulin and albumin: Development during the newborn period. J Pediatr 72:685–689, 1968
98. Taylor B, Norman AP, Orgel HA, et al.: Transient IgA deficiency and pathogenesis of infantile atopy. Lancet 2:111–113, 1973
99. Roy CC, Dubois RS: The human gut and immune homeostasis. Clin Pedatr 10:275–281, 1971
100. Taylor KB: Alimentary and gastrointestinal allergy. Front Gastrointest Res 1:1–11, 1975
101. Kaufman HS, Hobbs JR: Immunoglobulin deficiencies in an atopic population. Lancet 2:1061–1063, 1970
102. Harrison M, Kilby A, Walker-Smith JA, et al.: Cow's milk protein intolerance: A possible association with gastroenteritis, lactose intolerance, and IgA deficiency. Br Med J 1:1501–1504, 1976
103. Fineman SM, Rosen FS, Geha RS: Transient hypogammaglobulinemia, elevated immunoglobulin E levels and food allergy. J Allergy Clin Immunol 64:216–222, 1979
104. Buckley RH, Dees SC: Correlation of milk precipitins with IgA deficiency. N Engl J Med 281:465–469, 1969
105. Amman AJ, Hong R: Anti antiserum antibody as a cause of double precipitin rings in immunoglobulin quantitation and its relation to milk precipitins. J Immunol 106:567–569, 1971
106. Cunningham-Rundles C, Brandeis WE, Good RA, et al.: Milk precipitins, circulating immune complexes, and IgA deficiency. Proc Natl Acad Sci 75:3387–3389, 1978
107. Barrett DJ, Bertani L, Ware DW, et al.: Milk precipitins in selective IgA deficiency. Ann Allergy 42:73–76, 1979
108. Vendel S: Cow's milk idiosyncrasy in infants. Acta Paediatr (Suppl 5) 35:3–37, 1948
109. Coombs RRA, Gell PGH: Classification of allergic reactions responsible for clinical hypersensitivity and disease, in Gell PGH, Coombs RRA, Lachman PJ (eds): Clinical Aspects of Immunology. London, Blackwell, 1975, p 761
110. Austin KF: Histamine and other mediators of allergic reactions, in Samter M, Alexander HL, Talmage DW, et al. (eds): Immunological Diseases, Boston, Little, Brown, 1965, pp 211–225.
111. Wide L, Bennich H, Johansson SGO: Diagnosis of allergy by an in-vitro test for allergen antibodies. Lancet 2:1105–1107, 1967
112. Shiner M, Ballard J, Brook CGD, et al.: Intestinal biopsy in the diagnosis of cow's milk protein intolerance without acute symptoms. Lancet 2:1060–1063, 1975
113. Wütrich B, Kopper E: Determination of specific IgE serum antibodies using the radio allergosorbent-test (RAST) and its significance for the diagnosis of atopic allergy. Schweiz Med Wochenschr 105:1337–1345, 1975
114. Parish WE: Detectin of reagins, IgG, IgA and IgM antibodies in human sera. Int Arch Allergy 36:245–265, 1969
115. May CD, Lyman M, Alberto R, et al.: Procedures for immunochemical study of histamine release from leukocytes with small volume of blood. J Allergy 46:12–20, 1970
116. Galant SP, Bullock J, Frick OL: An immunological approach to the diagnosis of food sensitivity. Clin Allergy 3:363–372, 1973

117. Parish WE: Release of histamine and slow reacting substance with mast cell changes after challenge with human lung sensitized passively with reagin in vitro. Nature (London) 215:738–739, 1967
118. Heiner DC, Rose B: A study of antibody responses by radioimmunodiffusion with demonstration of γD antigen-binding activity in four sera. J Immunol 104:691–697, 1970
119. Kilby A, Walker-Smith JA, Wood CBS: Small intestinal mucosa in cow's milk allergy. Lancet 1:531, 1975
120. Scherzer H, Ward PA: Lung and dermal vascular injury produced by preformed immune complexes. Am Rev Respir Dis 117:551–557, 1978
121. Stafford HA, Polmar SH, Boat TF: Immunologic studies in cow's milk-induced pulmonary hemosiderosis. Pediatr Res 11:898–903, 1977
122. Kravis T, Henson PM: Accumulation of platelets at sites of antigen-antibody-mediated injury: A possible role for IgE antibody and mast cells. J Immunol 118:1569–1573, 1977
123. Rubin MI: Allergic intestinal bleeding in newborn: Clinical syndrome. Am J Med Sci 200:385–390, 1940
124. Wilson JF, Heiner DC, Lahey ME: Milk-induced gastrointestinal bleeding in infants with hypochromic microcytic anemia. JAMA 189:122–126, 1964
125. Waldmann TA, Wochner RD, Laster L, et al.: Allergic gastroenteropathy: A cause of excessive gastrointestinal protein loss. N Engl J Med 276:761–769, 1967
126. Matsumura T, Kuroume T, Fukushima I: Significance of food allergy in the etiology of orthostatic albuminuria. J Asthma Res 3:325–329, 1966
127. Sandberg DH, McIntosh RM, Bernstein CW, et al.: Severe steroid-responsive nephrosis associated with hypersensitivity. Lancet 1:388–390, 1977
128. Carr RI, Andrist M, McDuffie F: Studies on the possibility of food induced immune-complex disease. Fed Proc 35:574, 1976
129. Penner E, Katz LA, Milgrom F: Microsomal antibody and circulating immune complexes in allergic gastroenteropathy. Lancet 1:669, 1978
130. May CD, Alberto R: In-vivo stimulation of peripheral lymphocytes to proliferation after oral challenge of children allergic to foods. Int Arch Allergy 43:525–532, 1972
131. Cooke RA: Protein derivatives as factors in allergy. Ann Intern Med 16:71–80, 1942
132. Spies JR, Stevan MA, Stein WJ, et al.: The chemistry of allergens. XX. New antigens generated by pepsin hydrolysis of bovine milk proteins. J Allergy 45:208–219, 1970
132. Haddad ZH, Kalra V, Verma S: IgE antibodies to pepetic and peptic-tryptic digests of betalactoglobulin: Significance in food hypersensitivity. Ann Allergy 42:368–371, 1979

5
Manifestations

Cow's milk allergy may be manifest in a wide variety of symptoms and signs, few of which can be considered pathognomonic of milk allergy. In fact, multiple system involvement has complicated the recognition of milk allergy, frequently causing misdiagnosis or confusion with other conditions. Symptoms vary from severe anaphylaxis to mild abdominal pain, and from immediate vomiting or diarrhea to delayed reactions such as chronic low-grade gastrointestinal blood loss, which may go unnoticed for months.

The frequency of different manifestations has varied from one report to another, being partly influenced by the investigator's case selection as well as by factors such as age, diagnostic criteria, and laboratory tests used. The gastrointestinal tract is the most frequently involved system, followed by the respiratory tract and skin, and then other body systems.

Multiple symptomatology is noted in more than one-half of the patients.[1-3] In the same patient, separate exposures occasionally lead to involvement of different shock organs and may be associated with varying latency periods, duration of symptoms, and severity of reaction. In general, however, the pattern of reaction manifest in a given patient is highly consistent compared with the pattern differences observed between individual patients. The data compiled by Lebenthal[4] from five studies[2,5-8] indicated that the presenting symptoms were diarrhea in 88 percent, vomiting in 44 percent, abdominal pain in 39 percent, atopic dermatitis in 33 percent, rhinitis in 31 percent, asthma in 31 percent, urticaria in 13 percent, and anaphylaxis in 12 percent.

In this chapter, we will consider the more common manifestations of cow's milk allergy. Several less common symptoms and signs reported in the literature also will be discussed briefly.

GASTROINTESTINAL MANIFESTATIONS

One would expect the gastrointestinal tract to be the shock organ most frequently involved in any food allergy, and this proves to be so. Overdiagnosis appears to be more frequent than underdiagnosis as viewed by most hospital-based academicians; they see many referred infants who have been labeled as being milk-sensitive without a firm basis for that diagnosis. Actually, as many or more infants with mild or delayed allergic reactions may go unrecognized. These factors contribute to the wide range in estimates of the prevalence of milk allergy. Gastrointestinal manifestations (Table 5-1) that have been attributed to cow's milk allergy, include the following:

1. *Vomiting.* Vomiting has been noted in one-fourth to one-half of patients with cow's milk allergy.[1-4, 9, 10] It usually occurs within one hour after the ingestion of milk, and the vomitus often contains a considerable amount of mucus. It may be severe, persisting and leading to dehydration and electrolyte imbalance. Occasionally, the infant presents with projectile vomiting that may be associated with abdominal distention simulating acute intestinal obstruction,[11, 12] or it may lead to a suspicion of hypertrophic pyloric stenosis.

   Sometimes milk-induced vomiting is associated with acetonemia, acetonuria, peculiar breath odor, pallor, tachycardia, and cerebral depression. This symptom-complex has been referred to as *acetonemic vomiting, recurrent vomiting with acetonuria,* or *cyclic vomiting of childhood.* In 25 (81 percent) of 31 patients with this syndrome, cow's milk alone, or in association with other food allergens, was believed responsible.[13]

2. *Abdominal pain.* Stomachache, vague abdominal pain, or colic may be encountered in about one-third of milk-sensitive patients.[1, 3, 8, 9, 14] In a series of 48 infants with colic, milk allergy was believed to be the chief cause in 12 percent and a contributing cause in another 19 percent.[15] During infancy, the picture is often that of prolonged crying and flexion of the thighs, which commonly occur during or shortly following feeding.

Table 5-1

Gastrointestinal Manifestations	
Vomiting	Protein-losing enteropathy
Abdominal pain	Enterocolitis
Diarrhea	Ulcerative colitis
Steatorrhea	Constipation
Malabsorption	Proctalgia
Intestinal bleeding	Refusal of milk
gross	Stomatitis
occult	Edema of lips

The infant may be a poor sleeper and awaken with apparent abdominal cramps that are not relieved by the usual remedies such as picking up, rubbing the back, placing him on his stomach, applying hot water bottles, or feeding him. The more cow's milk a milk-sensitive infant is fed, however, the more symptoms he exhibits. A frequent statement by the mother is: "As soon as he finishes his bottle he is hungry again, but after he takes a little more he starts to scream again." Occasionally, the clinical picture is difficult to differentiate from intussusception.[16, 17]

In older children, the pain is usually milder than it is in infants. It may be periumbilical, epigastric, or poorly localized. The relationship between symptoms and food allergy is often overlooked, particularly in patients in whom the reaction is of the delayed-onset type.

Allergic colic is frequently associated with or followed later by other allergic disorders,[18] and it has been considered by some authors to be a major component of a syndrome consisting of abdominal pain, headache, leg aches, fatigue, respiratory allergies, pallor, and nervous tension.[19-21]

3. *Diarrhea.* Diarrhea of various degrees is a common symptom of cow's milk allergy and has been noted in one-fourth to three-fourths of milk-sensitive patients.[1, 4, 9, 16, 22] The stools are frequent and loose; they are yellow or green; they often contain excessive mucus; at times they may be streaked with visible blood; they may be watery or curdled; and they often cause irritation to the perianal region. Secondary (milk-induced) lactase deficiency is not uncommon.[23]

Allergic diarrhea may be mild and disappear within a few days or it may be prolonged and intractable.[24, 25] Severe or protracted diarrhea often is accompanied by damaged intestinal mucosa, dehydration, electrolyte imbalance, malabsorption, weight loss, and a wide variety of transient food intolerances. An allergic cause is seldom considered at the onset and may not be recognized before several weeks or months have elapsed, or until there have been several prolonged recurrences without evidence of an infectious cause.

4. *Steatorrhea.* One manifestation of gastrointestinal milk allergy may be decreased absorption of fat, resulting in bulky fatty stools, abdominal distention, and poor growth.[5] The xylose tolerance test is frequently abnormal, indicating diffuse jejunal mucosal involvement. It becomes normal on milk-free diet and subnormal on reintroduction of milk.[26] On milk challenge, the percentage of ingested fat in the stools may rise to more than 10 times the percentage noted during avoidance of cow's milk.[23] Steatorrhea caused by milk allergy is most frequent during childhood but also can occur in adults.[27, 28]

5. *Malabsorption of other nutrients.* In addition to malabsorption of fat, other nutrients such as carbohydrates, proteins, and fat-soluble vitamins may be poorly absorbed, resulting in growth retardation and symptoms of

malnutrition. Undigested dietary constituents are often observed in the stool. The clinical picture and histologic changes in the intestinal mucosa may resemble those of other conditions causing malabsorption. Marked improvement, however, occurs on a milk-free diet, and a recurrence is produced by milk challenge.[10, 29] The insult to the intestinal mucosa is often reflected as a decrease in the mucosal disaccharidase activity or in D-xylose absorption.[26]

Malabsorption of minerals, such as calcium and zinc, may combine with intrinsic peculiarities of milk to produce dramatic symptoms. The high phosphate content of cow's milk can lead to neonatal tetany as a result of a decreased absorption of calcium. This is more likely to occur, even in older infants, when there is excessive loss of calcium from the gastrointestinal tract as a result of milk allergy. Cow's milk has a lower content of zinc than human milk, and in the presence of milk-related malabsorption, zinc deficiency may cause a syndrome called acrodermatitis enteropathica (See Chap. 7).

Radiographic studies with barium swallow may show hasty passage through the proximal small intestine after milk ingestion compared with slower passage in similar studies while on a milk-free diet.[30] Such an abnormality not only may prevent the ingested food from remaining in the jejunum the normal period of time required for digestion and absorption, but it also compromises the ability of the mucosa to digest each gram of food per unit of time it is in contact with the mucosal surface.

6. *Intestinal bleeding.* Intestinal bleeding is a relatively common manifestation of cow's milk allergy that is often misdiagnosed. The bleeding may be gross and easily noticed by the parents, or occult and unnoticed for long periods.

   (a) *Gross bleeding.* This manifestation of cow's milk allergy was first described by Rubin.[31] It occurs usually during the first few weeks of life. The stools are intermixed with blood that varies in quantity from barely perceptible discoloration to profuse bleeding. There is usually excessive mucus, and the stools are often loose. Proctoscopy may reveal a red, friable, and ulcerated mucosa that bleeds easily.[16]

   The condition usually improves within two days of elimination of milk from the diet and after a few months of a milk-free diet, milk can often be reintroduced without apparent ill effect.

   (b) *Occult bleeding.* This type of bleeding occurs usually in infants 3 to 12 months of age as a chronic form of low-grade blood loss. It may result in profound anemia in spite of an adequate dietary intake of iron. The relation to cow's milk allergy was first suspected by Wilson et al.,[32] in a group of infants with iron-deficiency anemia. These workers noted occult gastrointestinal bleeding in 40 percent, circulating precipitins to cow's milk in more than 75 percent, and the presence of serum proteins in the fasting gastric juice in 12 out of 13 anemic infants tested. Later, the same authors documented the association between the gastrointestinal bleeding and the ingestion of homogenized whole cow's milk.[33] The fecal blood loss was quantitatively determined by infusing ^{51}Cr-labeled autologous erythrocytes and measuring the total radioactivity appearing in the stools.[34] The loss varied between 0.6 and 10.3 ml of blood per day, with a profound decrease on elimination of homogenized whole cow's milk and the substitution of either heat-treated milk or soybean formulas (Fig. 5-1). A direct relationship was noted between the amount of ingested whole cow's milk and the amount of fecal blood loss (Fig. 5-2). The precipitating antibodies were largely directed toward heat-labile proteins in cow's milk, and boiling of milk reduced or eliminated the intestinal blood loss in at least some of the children. Infants with this syndrome did poorly on regular homogenized pasteurized cow's milk, but thrived on a milk substitute and usually on heat-treated (boiled or evaporated) cow's milk. Follow-up of several of these infants suggested that milk-induced bleeding seldom persists beyond the age of 2 years.

7. *Gastrointestinal protein loss.* A form of cow's milk-induced "allergic gastroenteropathy" has been described by Waldmann et al.[35] The syndrome consists of edema, growth retardation, severe hypoalbuminemia, hypogammaglobulinemia, anemia, and milk precipitins in the serum. An increase in the number of eosinophils was noted in the circulation, intestinal mucosa, and stools. There was a striking response to elimination of milk from the diet or to corticosteroid therapy. The rate of albumin synthesis was normal or increased but its half-life was markedly shortened with a range between 2.8 and 3.9 days, compared with a mean of 17 days in controls. Gastrointestinal loss of protein was demonstrated by greatly increased fecal excretion of intravenously administered ^{131}I-polyvinylpyrrolidone or ^{51}Cr-albumin. Similar findings were reported by Lebenthal et al.,[8] who described three patients with the syndrome in whom the offending protein was beta-lactoglobulin.

8. *Enterocolitis.* Acute enterocolitis is mainly a disease of neonates, with an increased incidence in low-birth-weight infants or in the presence of other illness such as sepsis or hypoxia. The infant is usually seriously ill and has vomiting, abdominal distention, bloody stools, and may have a characteristic radiologic appearance of air in the intestinal wall (pneumatosis intestinalis), mainly in the ileum and colon. The pathogenesis is not well understood, but precipitating factors may include ischemia, infection, hyperosmolarity of oral feedings, and altered host defenses.[36,37] In 1973, cow's milk intolerance was reported to be involved in a case of acute necrotizing enterocolitis.[38] Since then, additional cases have been reported.[39-41] In addition to the precipitation of the above syndrome after milk challenge, Powell[40] demonstrated a rise of more than 4,000/cu mm in the circulating polymorphonuclear leukocyte count at 6 to 8 hours postchallenge.

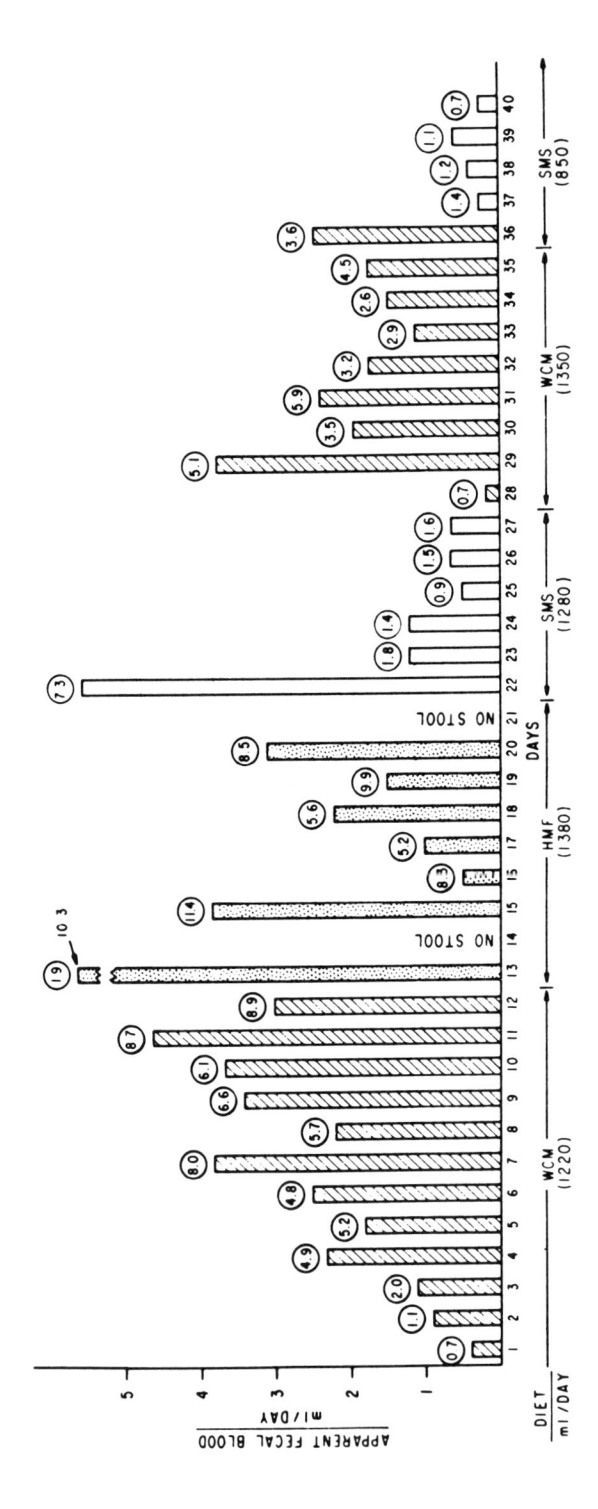

Fig. 5-1. Milk-induced fecal blood loss in a 13-month-old infant. Circles atop the vertical bars refer to the concentration of blood in milliliters per 100 gm of stool. (WCM, whole cow's milk; HFM, heat-modified milk formula; SMS, soya milk substitute). From Wilson JF, Lahey ME, Heiner DC: Studies on iron metabolism. V. Further observations on cow's milk-induced gastrointestinal bleeding in infants with iron-deficiency anemia. J Pediatr 84:335-344, 1974. Reproduced with permission.

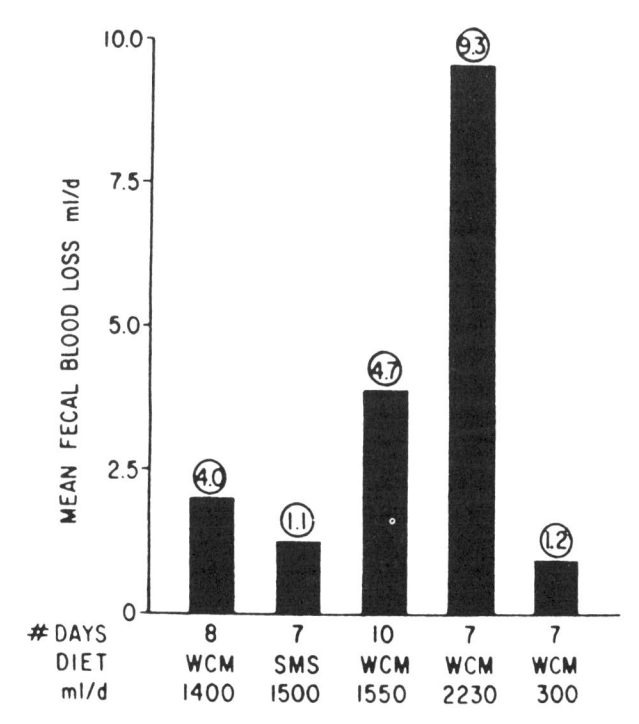

Fig. 5-2. Relationship between the amount of whole cow's milk ingested and the degree of fecal blood loss during consecutive periods in a 25-month-old infant. (WCM, whole cow's milk; SMS, Soya milk substitute.) From Wilson JF, Lahey ME, Heiner DC: Studies on iron metabolism. V. Further observations on cow's milk-induced gastrointestinal bleeding in infants with iron deficiency anemia. J Pediatr 84:335-344, 1974. Reproduced with permission.

9. *Ulcerative colitis.* Ulcerative colitis is a chronic inflammatory condition in which acute exacerbations are often related to intolerance to specific foods. Milk has been implicated rather frequently.[42,43] In patients with ulcerative colitis, the incidence of cow's milk feeding from the first month of life was twice that in controls.[44] An increase in circulating antibodies to milk was noted in some patients but not in others, and there was little relationship between the level of antibodies and the severity of the condition.[45-47] Nevertheless, ulcerative colitis may be associated with a variety of food allergies, autoantibodies, and antibodies to intestinal bacteria or to circulating endotoxin. Eosinophilia in the peripheral blood and in the rectal and colonic mucosa is common. Response to the oral administration of disodium cromoglycate is frequently favorable,[48] suggesting that immediate hypersensitivity and chemical mediator release from mast cells may play a role in the pathogenesis. Probably infections, hypersensitivity to

ingested foods, and a propensity to autoimmunity can each play a contributory role.
10. *Constipation.* Constipation may be a manifestation of milk allergy.[1,9,22,49] Stools may be hard, resulting in painful defecation. The addition of juices, malt, or Karo syrup to the formula may sometimes help. More often, laxatives, enemas, or suppositories are used until the parent or physician discovers that the most effective measure is a sharp decrease or total elimination of cow's milk from the diet. Occasionally, in infants with gastrointestinal milk allergy, periods of constipation alternate with periods of diarrhea.[50]
11. *Proctalgia.* Proctalgia was thought to be caused by milk allergy in an infant who had had painful defecation for several months but had not had any constipation.[17] There was a bilateral family history of allergy. Proctoscopy revealed a slight redundance of the rectosigmoid mucosa without apparent organic cause. The infant improved within 3 days after cow's milk had been eliminated from the diet. The symptoms recurred after oral milk challenge. Several months later the infant appeared able to tolerate cow's milk although he developed respiratory allergy.
12. *Refusal of milk.* Loss of appetite for cow's milk or refusal of the milk bottle is not uncommon in milk-sensitive children.[1,22] This phenomenon may be the sole symptom or may occur in association with other evidences of milk allergy.[51] When cow's milk is eliminated and a milk substitute such as soybean formula is provided, the child's appetite improves and he or she often has a more adequate weight gain.
13. *Stomatitis.* In some patients, itching or burning in the mouth has been attributed to local contact with cow's milk. The condition may be associated with multiple superficial ulcerations in the oral mucosa.[52] The role of cow's milk in allergic stomatitis is probably less than that of other food allergens such as chocolate, apples, citrus fruits, tomatoes, pineapple, bananas, and walnuts.[49]
14. *Edema of lips.* Occasionally, a patient's lips and tongue swell from contact with milk. The edema usually develops within minutes after contact and disappears spontaneously within hours if further exposure does not occur.

Mucosal Morphology and Enzyme Abnormalities

HISTOLOGIC STUDIES

In patients having colitis-like symptoms, sigmoidoscopy may show a hemorrhagic, friable mucosa with ulcerations. Mucosal biopsy reveals nonspecific changes varying from a slight infiltrate of lymphocytes and plasma cells in the lamina propria to polymorphonuclear cell infiltrate, destruction of surface epithelium, crypt abscesses, and distortion of rectal glands. After milk elimination, the

Manifestations

mucosa reverts to normal within a few days to a few weeks.[16] Eosinophils have infiltrated the rectal mucosa after a milk enema.[53]

In children presenting with malabsorption, the mucosal changes involve mainly the proximal small intestine.[30] The small bowel biopsy specimen frequently appears normal by light microscopy,[54, 55] but that appearance may be owing to a patchy pattern of the lesion. A wide variety of changes, however, have been reported in the literature. Dissecting microscopy has revealed a variety of nonspecific histologic changes that may be induced by milk ingestion but that often do not correlate very well with the intensity of symptoms.[10, 35, 56-60] In fact a significant milk-induced intestinal pathologic condition is not always accompanied by symptoms, and one therefore often cannot adequately judge improvement purely on the basis of dissolution of symptoms. With the patient on a milk-free diet, in most cases the mucosa will return to a normal state within a few months, and occasionally in several months.

The histologic appearance may correspond to one of the following: (1) *Slight changes*. The villi are broadened or branched but not shortened, and there is a slight increase in the cellular density of the lamina propria. (2) *Partial villous atrophy*. The villi are short and separated by tortuous ridges, giving the mucosa a convoluted appearance. The villous epithelium contains increased numbers of goblet cells. The lamina propria shows a cellular infiltrate of plasma cells, eosinophils, and lymphocytes. There also may be an increase in mast cells. (3) *Subtotal villous atrophy*. There is a flat mucosa, often with a mosaic pattern, and even more marked chronic inflammatory changes.

Similar mucosal changes may be seen in patients with celiac disease, soybean intolerance, certain disaccharidase deficiencies, transient exudative enteropathy, acute gastroenteritis, and prolonged nonspecific enterocolitis.[55, 58, 61, 62] Several recent investigations[60, 63, 64] have shown increased numbers of mast cells, eosinophils, and intraepithelial lymphocytes in the mucosal biopsies of subjects with food allergies. Degranulation of mast cells occurred after challenge with the specific food allergen. Treatment with oral disodium cromoglycate results in normalization of the mucosa in some subjects and may prevent changes after challenge with the food allergen.

DISACCHARIDASE ACTIVITY

In the presence of milk-related symptoms, jejunal mucosal specimens frequently show depressed activities of the disaccharidase enzymes lactase, sucrase, maltase, and palatinase.[60, 62] Normalization of enzyme activities may not be attained until after several weeks of a milk-free diet, and improved enzyme activity does not always parallel improvement in histologic findings.[62, 65]

IMMUNOFLUORESCENCE STUDIES

Savilahti[66] carried out immunologic studies on the small intestinal mucosa after milk challenge and noted an increase in the numbers of IgA- and IgM-containing cells, even in patients who did not exhibit clinical relapse. He found little evidence for the involvement of IgE or complement in the reaction. On the other hand, Shiner et al.[57, 67] also studied jejunal mucosal changes before and after milk challenge in four infants suspected of having milk allergy but who had no symptoms on challenge. Mucosal biopsies in two showed morphologic and immunologic changes as well as evidence of serum complement activation after the milk challenge. Immunofluorescence revealed an increase in the mucosa of IgG, IgA, IgM, IgE, and complement, to various degrees in individual patients. Electron microscopy showed vacuolation and mitochondrial swelling in the villous epithelium with widening of the subepithelial connective tissue spaces. Eosinophils, degranulated mast cells, and macrophages had increased in number, and plasma cells showed dilated cysternae, suggesting increased immunoglobulin production. Harris et al.,[68] however, noted little difference in the IgG-, IgA-, or IgM-containing plasma cells in the lamina propria of infants with milk-induced colic, whether the infants were off cow's milk feedings or on them, but the number of IgE-plasma cells was strikingly higher after milk challenge compared with the number at prechallenge. Such increases in IgE-bearing plasma cells is not specific for milk allergy because it may occur with other conditions associated with mucosal damage, including celiac disease and bacterial gastroenteritis.[69] Other workers have noted individual variations in the findings by immunofluorescence during studies of the jejunal mucosa after oral milk challenge.[29]

RESPIRATORY MANIFESTATIONS

The respiratory tract is probably the second most common target system for hypersensitivity to cow's milk. Symptoms vary from mild rhinorrhea to severe pulmonary disease, as shown below, and in Table 5-2. Most milk-induced respiratory symptoms are IgE-mediated. In chronic pulmonary disease, however, immune-complex and cell-mediated reactions seem to predominate.

1. *Rhinitis.* Nasal stuffiness, paroxysmal sneezing, and persistent watery or mucoid discharge have been noted in 10 to 30 percent of children with cow's milk allergy.[1-4, 9, 70] The symptoms frequently date from the first few weeks of life, and they commonly begin a few days or weeks after the cow's milk formula feeding has been started. The child may have breathing difficulty, particularly during sleep, or an irritating cough associated with a postnasal

Table 5-2

Respiratory Manifestations	
Rhinitis	Recurrent pneumonia
Chronic cough	Pulmonary hemosiderosis
Bronchitis	Upper airway obstruction
Asthma	Serous otitis media

drip. The nasal mucosa usually appears edematous and pale, and has a thin mucoid discharge. A nasal smear may show increased eosinophils. A bluish discoloration of the lower eyelids ("allergic shiners") may develop. In older children frequent rubbing of the nose may produce a transverse crease on the nasal bridge.

2. *Chronic cough.* The terms *chest cold* or *congestion in the chest* are frequently mentioned by the mothers of children who have a chronic cough. The cough is frequently associated with noisy breathing and excessive mucus in the throat, and sometimes parents worry that their child is "gagging." Such symptoms were presenting complaints in 17 percent of 206 infants with cow's milk allergy.[1] Hypersecretion of mucus seems to be a predominant factor. In the absence of secondary infection, the child is usually afebrile and does not look impressively sick. There may be excessive mucus in the posterior pharynx, and auscultation usually reveals coarse rhonchi over the middle part of the chest and along the the trachea. In uncomplicated cases, the chest roentgenogram shows clear lung fields. Such affected children are frequently diagnosed as having upper respiratory infection, viral illness, bronchitis, bronchiolitis, bronchopneumonia, or pneumonia. Accordingly, they may be given unnecessary medications, including cough syrups, decongestants, or antibiotics. Relief, however, is not satisfactory until cow's milk is eliminated from the diet.

3. *Bronchitis.* Bronchitis is usually an ill-defined term in pediatric practice and is frequently mentioned as a diagnosis during respiratory illnesses. In milk-sensitive children, recurrent bronchitis was recorded as the presenting symptom in 79 out of 150 (53 percent) in one series,[71] in 5 out of 17 (29 percent) in another,[72] and in 10 out of 59 (17 percent) in a third.[3] The respiratory symptoms may take the form of intermittent attacks of cough, dyspnea, tachypnea, and occasionally fever. The condition is recurrent and frequently requires hospitalization. Investigations for cystic fibrosis, aspiration of a foreign body, an immunodeficiency disease, or other explanations have negative results, and recurrent bronchitis appears to be the most fitting diagnosis. Symptomatic treatment results in a temporary improvement, but dramatic relief occurs on a milk-free diet. A familial tendency was noted by Gerrard.[73] In some patients, increased titers of hemagglutinating antibodies to milk were detected.[74]

4. *Asthma.* Bronchial asthma has been noted in 7 to 29 percent of milk-sensitive children. [1, 3, 9, 22, 71, 72] Narrowing of the large airways by bronchospasm and excessive bronchial secretion results in various degrees of wheezing, which is frequently loud enough to cause parental anxiety. An irritating cough may precede or accompany the wheezing. Between asthma attacks, the child is seldom completely symptom-free, and auscultation of the chest usually reveals scattered rhonchi, prolonged expiration, or mild wheezing.

Milk-related wheezing commonly begins early in life shortly after institution of feedings containing cow's milk. Recurrences are frequent, yet the cause-and-effect relationship is usually unrecognized for long periods. Many physicians are under the impression that asthma is rare in infants and are hesitant to diagnose asthma during infancy, not realizing that the peak of onset is under 1 year of age.[75, 76] We have seen many children with recurrent wheezing that has begun during the first few weeks of life and who required frequent emergency room visits, even multiple hospitalizations, until elimination of cow's milk from the diet resulted in complete disappearance of the asthma. After such a dramatic change, it is understandable that some parents resist subjecting the child to an oral milk challenge test. Nevertheless, our practice is to explain from the beginning the need for verification by a challenge test, and good cooperation is usually obtained.

5. *Recurrent pneumonia.* In 1958-1959, Heiner and Sears[77] noted that hypersensitivity to cow's milk could result in recurrent pneumonia as well as additional symptoms, which together comprised a syndrome.

Milk-induced Syndrome with Pulmonary Disease
Chronic or recurrent pulmonary disease
Allergic rhinitis, otitis media, cough, wheezing, or hemoptysis
Anorexia, vomiting, colic, or diarrhea
Failure to thrive
Iron deficiency anemia
Recurrent or persistent eosinophilia
Serum precipitins to multiple constituents of cow's milk

There was a close association between the syndrome and multiple precipitins to cow's milk proteins in the serum. The syndrome was later observed by other authors.[78-81] This syndrome must be suspected when precipitins to bovine milk proteins are found in sera of children with unexplained recurrent or chronic pulmonary disease who are fed cow's milk in any form. Screening large numbers of "allergic" children is much less rewarding. In children with milk allergy, the incidence of milk-related pulmonary infiltrates is probably less than 5 percent.[81]

The originally described group[77, 82, 83] comprised 7 children aged 6 weeks to 15 months with idiopathic chronic pulmonary disease, in whose sera precipitating antibodies to cow's milk were detectable by micro-Ouchterlony technique. Precipitins were directed to five or more consitituents of cow's milk and precipitates could be obtained when the sera were diluted 8- to 128-fold. All seven had a history of ingesting raw or pasteurized homogenized cow's milk, and all had chronic cough, recurrent fever, tachypnea, wheezes, and rales. The roentgenologic findings in the lungs consisted of changing patchy infiltrates, frequently associated with localized atelectasis, consolidation, peribronchial infiltrate, hilar adenopathy, pleural thickening, and reticular density (Fig. 5-3). Associated clinical findings included rhinitis, frequent otitis media, hemoptysis, gastrointestinal symptoms (vomiting, colic, anorexia, diarrhea), poor weight gain, eosinophilia, and profound anemia with hemoglobin ranging between 2.9 and 8.8 gm/dl. Most symptoms improved strikingly within a few days after the patient's diet was changed to a milk free one or to heat-treated milk (boiled or evaporated). The chest roentgenogram, however, may not clear for several weeks.

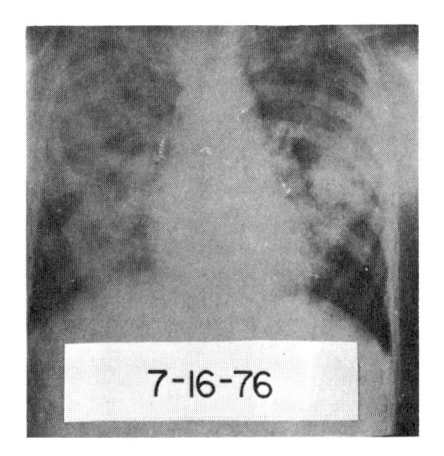

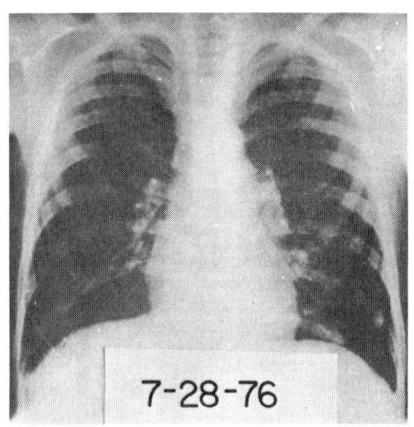

Fig. 5-3. Chronic patchy infiltrate in the lungs of a child whose serum showed multiple precipitins to cow's milk proteins. Resolution in the infiltrate was remarkable within 12 days after instituting a milk-free diet.

These patients had a positive intradermal test reaction to raw cow's milk but the control subjects did not. It is essential to use freshly prepared milk samples in dilutions greater than those that cause skin reactions in control subjects. Experience has subsequently shown that even with these precations the test results will occasionally be positive in apparently healthy children, and at times, negative in affected patients.

Reaginic antibodies do not seem to play a large role in the pathogenesis of pulmonary disease in this syndrome, although immune complexes may be involved and their deposition may be favored by the presence of reaginic antibodies (See Chap. 4). In the studies reported by Holland et al.,[79] less than five precipitate bands were detected. Our experience has also shown that many subjects with milk-related pulmonary symptoms have precipitins to less than five milk constituents and in titers of only 1:1 to 1:8. Such findings, however, are also much more frequent in control populations. The proportion of false positive results is greater and false negative results are less if this range of precipitins and titers is used as a diagnostic criterion.

The passive hemagglutination test has been used also in detecting similar antibodies.[74] In our hands, however, the precipitation test in agar is easier to perform, more reproducible, and it correlates better with symptoms.

The possible contribution of milk aspiration to pulmonary disease in this syndrome must be considered, particularly when vomiting and regurgitation are prominent features of the history. Since this point was not investigated in the first group of patients studied by Heiner and co-workers,[77, 83] the role of aspiration in those children is uncertain. In another group of 6 patients, however, in whom the clinical history led to a suspicion of aspiration, study of swallowing function by cineradiography showed aspiration of contrast media into the trachea in three patients.[81] In a group of children with chronic asthma and recurrent pneumonia studied by Euler et al.,[84] dysfunction of the lower esophageal sphincter was a frequent finding. Nevertheless, many symptoms of the above-mentioned syndrome cannot be explained by aspiration alone, since symptoms of some patients with pulmonary infiltrates clear on simple substitution of a soy formula that should also be aspirated. Nasal and ear symptoms also clear dramatically, and it is hard to see how aspiration alone could lead to nasal symptoms. Perhaps a slight or moderate amount of milk aspiration in an infant prone to hypersensitivity to bovine antigens could heighten his degree of sensitivity. His chances for developing all aspects of the syndrome may be greater than those of an infant of similar predisposition who did not aspirate or of an infant who aspirated but was not sensitive.

6. *Pulmonary hemosiderosis.* In pulmonary hemosiderosis, the iron-containing pigment, hemosiderin (an iron hydroxide-protein complex), accumulates in the lung parenchyma as a result of bleeding from alveolar capillaries. Such bleeding may result from an elevated pulmonary venous pressure because of a cardiac or vascular lesion (secondary pulmonary hemosiderosis) or, more commonly in children, it may occur without any abnormality in the pulmonary venous system (primary pulmonary hemosiderosis).[85-87]

The patient with active disease often presents with a pneumonia-like picture, hemoptysis, and a falling hematocrit. In some instances, however, the onset is insidious and may be without hemoptysis or anemia. Occasionally, the chest roentgenogram is normal for months or years during remissions, even though many iron-laden macrophages are found.

The diagnosis must be verified by detecting iron-laden macrophages in smears from tracheal aspirates or from the morning gastric washings (Fig. 5-4). Since infants and young children tend to swallow sputum, a satisfactory specimen is often difficult to obtain. Rarely, lung biopsy is needed to confirm the diagnosis. We prefer a small open biopsy under general anesthesia, since severe bleeding can occasionally follow needle biopsy done under local anesthesia.

In most cases of primary pulmonary hemosiderosis in older children,

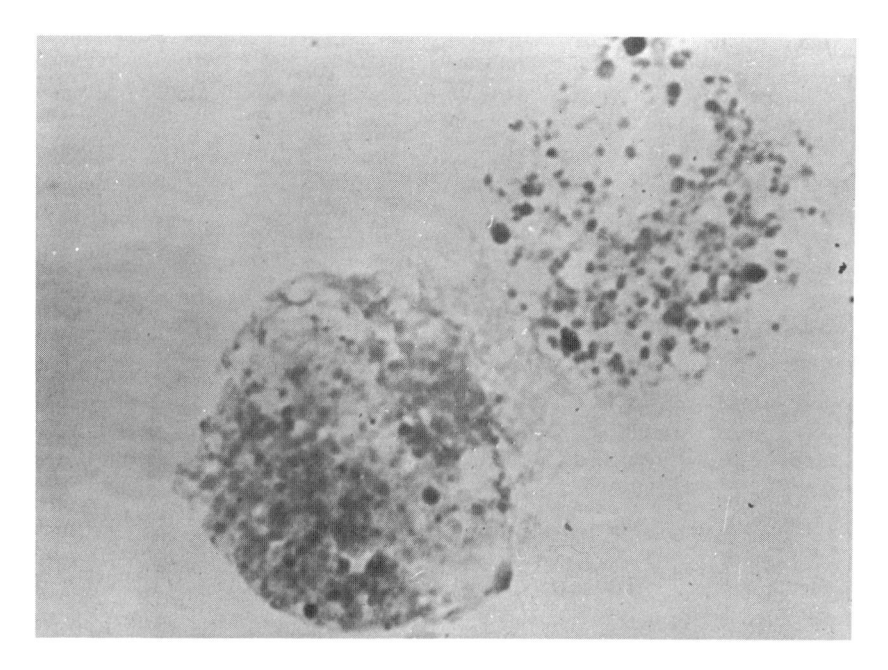

Fig. 5-4. Iron-laden macrophages in the gastric washing from a child with cow's milk-induced pulmonary hemosiderosis. The smear was stained with Prussian blue, which clearly demonstrates the diffuse cytoplasmic hemosiderin deposits in these cells.

no cause is obvious. In some cases, particularly during infancy, the cause is definitely related to the ingestion of cow's milk.

Four of the seven patients with chronic pulmonary disease and multiple milk precipitins described by Heiner et al.[83] had hemoptysis and were shown to have iron-laden macrophages in the bronchial or gastric aspirates. Eliminating cow's milk from the diet improved the symptoms, cleared the lungs, and improved the anemia. Boat and co-workers[88] described 6 children with milk-induced pulmonary hemosiderosis, in whom the pulmonary infiltrate was manifest within the first 6 months of life and was recurrent. No immunoglobulin deficiencies or evidence of recurrent aspiration was detected, although precipitins to cow's milk proteins were found.

Milk-induced primary pulmonary hemosiderosis probably occurs in about 10 percent of children with milk-related pulmonary infiltrates. It should be suspected whenever a young child who drinks cow's milk has recurrent pneumonia, hemoptysis, and anemia, especially when other allergic reactions are evident, such as rhinitis, wheezing, otitis media, or gastrointestinal symptoms. If there are precipitins to cow's milk proteins, the infant should certainly be given a trial of a milk-free diet for 4 to 6 weeks. Even in the absence of precipitins, a milk-free diet may be worth trying, since some such children seem to do well with this measure alone. If the child does not improve on a milk-free diet, or if aspiration as a contributory factor is suspected, the child should be examined for gastroesopageal reflux or abnormalities in swallowing function that could lead to aspiration.

The pathogenesis of milk-induced pulmonary hemosiderosis is not completely understood. As mentioned earlier (Chap. 4), immune complex deposition or an Arthus-like phenomenon is a likely underlying reaction. Besides a high titer of circulating precipitating antibodies to milk, a positive 4-hour intradermal test to milk antigens is a frequent finding.[88, 89]

In immunofluorescence studies on lung biopsy specimens, Kniker[81] showed particulate and amorphous deposits of IgG, IgA, C3, fibrin, and bovine serum albumin diffusely scattered throughout the lung tissue, particularly between cells and within polymorphonuclear leukocytes. The detection of intermittently circulating bovine serum albumin suggested that immune complexes arrived via the circulation. Total serum IgE levels were elevated in some patients [88, 90] but not in others.[81, 89] An increase in circulating specific IgE antibodies to alpha-casein and bovine serum albumin was also noted.[81] IgE-mediated reactions may be responsible for the allergies that often accompany infantile pulmonary hemosiderosis or may be involved in the pathogenesis of pulmonary disease by facilitating immune complex disposition.[91-93] Probably a variety of immunopathologic mechanisms may be involved in milk-induced pulmonary hemosiderosis. A joint contribution by antibodies and lymphocyte-mediated immune responses[89] is quite possible.

7. *Upper airway obstruction.* Some patients with milk-induced chronic pulmonary disease have been found to have upper airway obstruction resulting from hypertrophied tonsils or adenoids, as described by Boat et at.[88] Of the 6 patients with milk-induced pulmonary hemosiderosis described by these authors, 3 had markedly enlarged adenoids, sleeping alveolar hypoventilation, hypercapnia and acidosis, pulmonary arterial hypertension, and even failure of the right side of the heart. These manifestations promptly reversed after adenoidectomy. In early stages of this complication, before upper airway obstruction is severe and pulmonary hypertension is well established, a milk-free diet alone may likely prevent the development of cor pulmonale.

8. *Serous otitis media.* In serous or secretory otitis media, serous or mucoid fluid accumulates in the middle ear and may cause increased pressure and dysfunction of the middle-ear structures. Hearing loss is the most common serious complication. In young infants, serous otitis often is not discovered before superimposed secondary infection occurs and acute otitis media develops. The latter responds to antibiotic therapy, only to recur with the next respiratory infection. Older children may complain of pain or popping sensations in their ears and varying degrees of hearing impairment. In early stages, the tympanic membranes often appear full or bulging and have poor

mobility. A fluid level or air bubbles may be seen behind the tympanic membrane, and the light reflex is commonly distorted or absent. In longstanding cases, the tympanic membranes are thickened, may be retracted, dull and discolored, and often have white patches. Their extreme immobility, and the increased viscosity of the retained middle-ear fluid have lead to the term *glue ears.* Tympanometry often reveals a poor compliance of the tympanic membrane.

Etiologically, there appears to be no single causative factor responsible for serous otitis.[94] Secretory otitis media is probably seldom caused by a lack of secretory IgA, since the latter was detected in more than 60 percent of ear aspirates from patients with serous otitis.[95, 96] IgA deficiency may be a contributing factor, however, particularly in children who lack both serum and secretory IgA, or who have more severe forms of dysgammaglobulinemia or agammaglobulinemia.

Serous otitis media occurs with increased frequency in atopic children. With the control of other manifestations of allergy, the otitis significantly improved both clinically and by audiometry in 80 percent.[97] Clearly, allergy may play an important role. Food allergy should always be considered, and the physician should realize that milk allergy may be a major factor, particularly during the first two years of life, but occasionally in the older child or adult as well. A role for milk allergy in serous otitis is stressed by some[50] yet denied by others.[98] The mucosa of the eustachian tube and middle ear probably responds with allergic reactions in a manner similar to the response of the nasal mucosa. Blockage of the eustachian tube can cause negative pressure in the middle ear and result in accumulation of serous fluid. Increased mucosal secretory activity may be equally or more important. The condition may be largely the result of nasal allergy causing eustachian tube blockage or it may be primarily a problem of mucosal allergy in the eustachian tube and middle ear (allergic tubotympanitis).[99] Both may play a role in many instances. Rather ill-defined at present are the precise mechanisms leading to allergic serous otitis media, including the roles for specific immunoglobulin classes, various inflammatory cells, chemical mediators, complement components, and lymphokines.

DERMATOLOGIC MANIFESTATIONS

Dermatologic manifestations of cow's milk allergy (Table 5-3) probably occur in one-half to three-fourths of milk-sensitive infants. They are less common in older children and adults.

1. *Atopic dermatitis.* In most studies, atopic dermatitis or eczema has been reported to be the most common single manifestation of cow's milk allergy, being

Table 5-3

Dermatologic Manifestations	
Atopic dermatitis	Perianal rash
Urticaria	Purpura
Angioedema	Dermatitis herpetiformis
Seborrheic rashes	Alopecia
Contact rash	

noted in about one-half or more of children with milk allergy.[2, 3, 14, 22, 70, 71] This may, however, be caused partly by the ease with which dermatologic changes can be observed by parents and physicians, and to the greater concern parents have over chronic skin rashes than they have over chronic rhinitis, for example. Cow's milk allergy was noted to be the cause of atopic dermatitis in 66 percent of 41 children under 2 years of age[70] and in 17 percent of 81 children under 5 years of age.[100] In infants, lesions appear largely on the cheeks, forehead, extensor surfaces of the extremitis, inguinal regions, and buttocks. They also occur, but with less frequency, on the flexor surfaces of extremities, the antecubital and popliteal fossae, the palms, and soles. In older children, the face remains frequently involved, together with the neck and flexor surfaces of the limbs. In adolescents and adults, the lesions have a strong propensity to involve the flexural aspects of the large joints, particularly the antecubital and popliteal fossae.

In the acute or subacute stages, the lesions consist of pruritic erythema with excoriations, papules, and vesicles. Improvement often can be seen within a few days of avoiding the offending allergen. In chronic cases, dryness, thickening, and lichenification become manifest, and significant improvement may require weeks rather than days. Hyperpigmentation or hypopigmentation is a common accompaniment of atopic eczema. Both are usually transient but sometimes are permanent sequelae.

2. *Urticaria.* Urticaria is a less frequent manifestation of cow's milk allergy than atopic dermatitis, and is more likely to occur in older children. It was noted in 1.5 to 12 percent of subjects with cow's milk allergy.[1, 2, 72] It may be the sole manifestation, occur together with other continuing symptoms, or appear as an acute component of a systemic anaphylactic reaction.

Pruritic wheals may appear suddenly and disappear within a few hours to a few days. If milk ingestion is causative, urticaria may not clear until milk is completely avoided. The possible etiologic role of cow's milk is often not considered as rapidly as that of other foods such as strawberries, shell fish, or nuts, which are less frequently ingested, allowing easier observations of cause and effect by parents or by the patient.

3. *Angioedema.* Angioedema often accompanies urticaria but may occur alone as localized swelling, particularly in areas rich in loose areolar tissue. In-

volvement of the gastrointestinal submucosa may cause vomiting, colic, or severe pain, simulating an acute abdominal problem. Such symptoms are quite alarming but usually resolve within a few hours if feedings are withheld.

4. *Seborrheic rashes.* In a series of 187 infants with seborrhea, cow's milk appeared to be an offending allergen in 68 percent;[101] however, the diagnosis of cow's milk allergy was not documented in the patients by challenge tests after the patients improved on a milk-elimination diet. During a 10- to 15-year follow-up of patients in the study, a variety of allergic manifestations appeared in two-thirds of the patients, atopic eczema being diagnosed in more than one-third. Further studies are needed to evaluate more precisely the role of food allergy in seborrheic dermatoses.

5. *Contact rash.* We, as well as others,[102,103] have observed various forms of contact urticaria to cow's milk. Blotchy erythema and wheals may develop within a few minutes wherever milk comes in contact with the skin. The rash generally disappears within a few hours in the absence of further contact. In some infants, the lesions are seen almost constantly around the mouth, chin, neck, and upper part of the chest. This manifestation of milk allergy is believed, in most cases, to represent an immediate-type hypersensitivity. In a few instances, it may be of the delayed-type hypersensitivity (lymphocyte-mediated), manifested as contact dermatitis that reaches its peak intensity 48 to 72 hours after exposure.

6. *Perianal rash.* In milk-sensitive infants, a perianal rash may be secondary to irritating diarrheal stools. A contact rash caused by undigested milk proteins in the stools may also occur. Although few firm data exist to indicate the relative importance of these two mechanisms, they are probably often concomitant and synergistic in their effect.

7. *Purpura.* Purpura and petechial rashes are rare manifestations of milk allergy. Milk-induced thrombocytopenic purpura[104,105] may be somewhat more common than milk-induced anaphylactoid or Henoch-Schönlein purpura.[72] One should be aware that such conditions may exist, since eliminating cow's milk feedings in such instances is a simple and effective therapeutic measure.

8. *Dermatitis herpetiformis.* The ingestion of cow's milk appeared to be the cause of dermatitis herpetiformis in a 30-year-old woman who had had a primary malabsorption syndrome for 3 years.[106] The malabsorption improved when the patient was on a gluten-free and almost milk-free diet. After an increase in the milk intake, gastrointestinal symptoms recurred and typical dermatitis herpetiformis developed. Vesicular lesions appeared on the back, knees, and elbows, and a biopsy showed subepidermal bullae and a cellular infiltrate in the corium with a preponderance of lymphocytes, but with some eosinophils. The lesions disappeared on milk elimination and repeatedly recurred on milk challenge.

This case report suggests that in certain hypersensitive subjects the complete malabsorption-dermatitis herpetiformis syndrome could result from the ingestion of cow's milk. Although the pathogenesis of this process is not known, malabsorption, subtotal atrophy of the jejunal mucosa, and dermatitis herpetiformis have repeatedly been shown to be precipitated in certain persons by the ingestion of wheat gluten. Cow's milk ingestion has also been shown to lead to malabsorption and partial villous atrophy.[10,57,58,107]

9. *Alopecia.* Total alopecia believed to be caused by hypersensitivity to cow's milk has been reported in one infant [107a] Because of gastrointestinal milk allergy, the infant was off cow's milk from 2 weeks of age, and when he was refed cow's milk at 9 months of age, a generalized eczematous rash appeared and within one week, totally lost the hair of his scalp, eyebrows and eyelashes.

HEMATOLOGIC MANIFESTATIONS

1. *Anemia.* An association between the ingestion of whole cow's milk and the development of severe iron deficiency anemia of infancy has been well known for many decades. The major problem was generally believed to be inadequate intake of iron in primarily milk-fed infants, perhaps with milk actually inhibiting iron absorption. In 1962, however, Wilson and his colleagues[32] noted in a series of infants and young children with iron deficiency anemia that the stools were guaiac-positive in 40 percent, and in more than 75 percent the serum contained precipitating antibodies to cow's milk protein. Later studies by the same authors, using infusions of ^{51}Cr-labeled autologous erythrocytes, revealed that milk-induced fecal blood loss was clearly greater while the infants were ingesting homogenized milk than during periods of ingestion of a soybean or heat-processed cow's milk formula.[33] The fecal blood loss generally ranged from 0.6 to 10.3 ml per day. Although gross blood or darkened stools could not be detected by visual examination, isotope studies conclusively demonstrated that intestinal bleeding was quantitatively related to the amount of milk ingested[34] (Fig. 5-2). In a retrospective study of selected subjects with gastrointestinal milk allergy reported by Gryboski,[1,6] all had what appeared to be milk-related fecal blood loss and hypochromic microcytic anemia. These patients often had colitis and grossly visible blood in the stools.

With many infants, the substitution of evaporated milk for pasteurized milk will considerably reduce or stop blood loss within a few days, whereas with others, the intake of cow's milk in any form may need to be markedly decreased or completely eliminated. With reintroduction of whole cow's milk, the bleeding rapidly recurs. In may instances in which blood is not grossly visible in the stools, weeks or months may elapse before significant anemia appears. In others, anemia may occur within a few days to a few weeks, depending on both the intake of iron and the degree of intestinal bleeding. The blood loss, however, may be small enough that anemia does not occur if the intake of iron is adequate and the compensatory increase in production of hemoglobin and erythrocytes keeps pace with the loss.[108] Unless milk is eliminated, iron therapy alone accomplishes only partial reparation, and the blood loss continues in spite of partial or temporary resolution of the anemia.

As mentioned before, hypochromic microcytic anemia is commonly manifested in children with milk-induced chronic pulmonary disease, especially if there is concomintant pulmonary hemosiderosis.[77, 83]

A search for occult bleeding should always be made; Wilson et al.[34] found occult blood in the stools of about one-half of infants and young children with iron deficiency anemia who were daily ingesting a liter or more of homogenized pasteurized cow's milk. In infants with respiratory symptoms or positive findings in chest roentgenograms, the possibility of bleeding into the lungs must also be considered. Milk-induced blood loss should be suspected in any infant drinking more than half a liter of milk daily in whom there is anemia without an obvious cause.

2. *Hypoproteinemia.* In the first group of children with iron deficiency anemia studied by Wilson et al.,[32] serum albumin ranged between 1.23 and 4.65 gm/100 ml with a mean value of 3.48 compared with 4.44 gm/100 ml for a control group. Gamma globulin values were similar in the two groups. Of 13 anemic children tested, 12 had serum proteins readily detectable in their gastric juice after fasting. Waldmann et al.[35] described more severe degrees of hypoproteinemia in children with milk-induced enteropathies. Isotope studies showed an association between gastrointestinal albumin loss and milk ingestion in some of the subjects. The assocation between ingestion of fresh cow's milk and protein loss in 12 infants with iron deficiency anemia was studied by Woodruff and Clark.[109] Intravenous injection of small quantities of ^{131}I-albumin followed by counts of whole-body radioactivity showed that 7 of the 12 patients had a rapid turnover of albumin, with a half-life range of 3.1 to 8.8 days and a mean of 6.4 days. A control group showed an albumin half-life range of 10.2 to 17.6 days with a mean of 12.6 days. Antibodies to cow's milk proteins were detected in the serum in 6 out of the 7 patients and in the stools of 3 out of 6. Correction of the anemia with parenteral iron therapy had no effect on the rapid albumin turnover, indicating that the gastrointestinal dysfunction was not caused by anemia per se. Feeding evaporated milk instead of fresh cow's milk lengthened the albumin half-life in four out of five patients, while feeding a soybean formula was followed by normalization of the values in each instance.

3. *Thrombocytopenia.* A reduction in the number of circulating platelets is a common finding in anaphylactic reactions.[110] In a group of adults with food allergy, ingestion of the offending allergen was followed within 90 minutes

by a reduction in the platelet count averaging 30 percent, but in many of the patients the change was not significant.[111, 112]

Osvath and Markus[113] studied hematologic changes before and during the 3 hours postchallenge in 35 children with milk and egg allergies. In 80 percent of patients, the platelet count was reduced by more than 35 percent, and the eosinophil count rose to greater than twofold. Nevertheless, some patients with pronounced allergic reaction to cow's milk had neither thrombocytopenia nor eosinophilia.

Jones[105] reported a case of a newborn boy with purpura and thrombocytopenia with platelet counts between 3,000 and 6,000/cu mm for 3 weeks; the platelet count rose dramatically when cow's milk formula was discontinued and clear liquids were fed. On resumption of the milk formula feeding, the platelet count dropped rapidly. On a milk-free diet, the infant was asymptomatic and the platelet count became normal (Fig. 5-5). When the child was 1 year old, the mother tried to reintroduce milk to the diet on two occasions, but each time the infant developed severe wheezing and easy bruising.

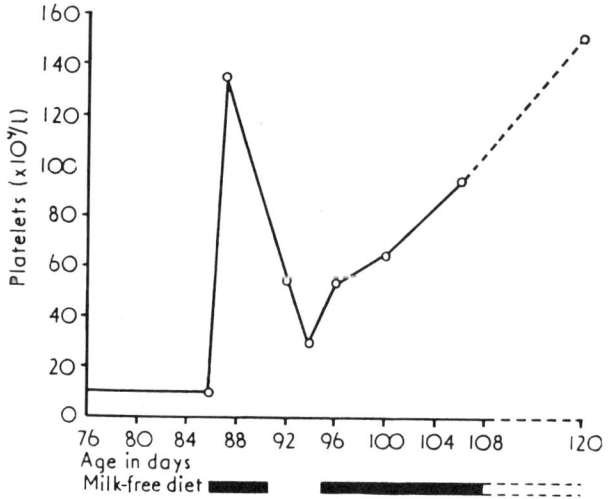

Fig. 5-5. Reversal of thrombocytopenia during milk-free diet, and recurrence with milk ingestion. From Jones RHT: Congenital thrombocytopenia and milk allergy. Arch Dis Child 52:744-745, 1977. Reproduced with permission.

Thrombocytopenia was reported by Whitfield and Barr[104] in a newborn girl with absent radius, severe vomiting, bloody diarrhea, and a platelet count of 25,000/cu mm. Her condition improved within a few days when she was given intravenous fluid and the milk formula was discontinued. Reintroduction of the formula resulted in increased symptoms and a drop in the platelet count to 16,000/cu mm. Dramatic clinical and hematologic improvement occurred when the infant was given a soybean formula and cow's milk was completely avoided. At 9 months, the infant tolerated a gradual reintroduction of cow's milk into the diet. The same authors reviewed reports on 40 cases of thrombocytopenia and absent radius (TAR syndrome) in the literature and found information suggesting cow's milk allergy in three.

4. *Eosinophilia.* In acute anaphylaxis, eosinophils rapidly shift from the circulation to the tissues and eosinopenia is usually noted. An increased number of circulating eosinophils, is commonly found in chronic atopic diseases. In patients with cow's milk allergy, between one-fouth and three-fourths have been considered to have eosinophilia.[10, 35, 56 58, 83, 88, 89] The eosinophilia usually disappears along with amelioration of symptoms after milk has been eliminated from the diet, and it recurs on provocation challenge.[8, 113, 114]

Unlike the previously mentioned hemotologic changes, i.e., anemia, hypoproteinemia, and thrombocytopenia, eosinophilia may well be beneficial. The eosinophil has a high content of both histamine and arylsufatase, which can inactivate histamine and slow reacting substance of anaphylasis (SRS-A), respectively. The eosinophil seems to have additional roles in the host defense mechanisms.[115]

CENTRAL NERVOUS SYSTEM MANIFESTATIONS

Allergy of the central nervous system has been discussed in the literature for many years.[1, 116-124] A wide variety of neurologic and behavioral symptoms (as listed on p. 68) have been reported. The subjectivity and nonspecificity of symptoms, as well as a lack of well-controlled studies, have led to skepticism in the medical profession regarding the role of allergy in central nervous system symptomatology. In some patients, electroencephalographic abnormalities have disappeared after suspected allergens were avoided.[125]

According to some authors, about one-fifth of children with cow's milk allergy have central nervous system disorders.[1, 2, 9] Elimination of cow's milk from the diet results in marked improvement of symptoms as well as of other associated manifestations of allergy. Nevertheless, neurologic and behavioral symptoms in a child with cow's milk allergy may be secondary to severe or chronic allergic responses in the other systems. Also, while considering an allergic cause for any of the symptoms, one must not overlook possible psychiatric and nonallergic organic causes.

The Allergic Tension-Fatigue Syndrome

The term *allergic tension-fatigue syndrome* was coined by Speer in 1954[19] to describe a chronic symptom complex involving a variety of motor and sensory complaints frequently associated with evidences of respiratory and gastrointestinal allergy. Other authors earlier reported similar symptoms, and their relationship to allergy was discussed by Randolph.[116] Some authors believe the syndrome to be a delayed-onset allergic disorder of the central nervous system caused by inhalants or ingestants but more often by foods, especially milk, chocolate, wheat, and corn.[20, 126-128] The onset is often insidious and symptoms may go unrecognized for years, with frequent visits to physicians, multiple investigational procedures, and ineffective medications. The diagnosis is often missed, both because of the subjectivity of symptoms and because of the lack of a reliable laboratory test. Various combinations of the following symptoms have been noted:

1. Nervous tension, anxiety, listlessness, inability to concentrate, lethargy, apathy, somnolence, irritability, restlessness, insomnia, depression, learning disorders, dependency, hyperkinesis, or other behavior problems.
2. Fatigue, easy tiredness, weakness, fainting, dizziness, or aches.
3. Headache that is intermittent and usually mild, but occasionally migraine in nature or severe enough to cause the patient to lie down.
4. Abdominal discomfort or pain that is epigastric or generalized and has no obvious relationship to meals. (It is usually mild but occasionally severe enough to awaken the child during the night.)
5. Musculoskeletal pains in the form of myalgia or arthralgia, more often in the legs and apt to occur during the night (growing pains).
6. Pale face with a sallow appearance, although anemia is usually absent. (The infraorbital regions may be puffy with dark bluish discoloration [allergic shiners] thought to result from impedance of the venous drainage by the edematous nasal mucosa.)
7. Respiratory allergies in the form of allergic rhinitis, serous otitis media, or asthma.

The true prevalence of this syndrome is unknown but it seems to be noted by some[20, 128] more often than by others. We have occasionally seen typical cases with a dramatic response to the correct elimination diet. A poor response is often noted in patients with multiple allergens where the recognition and elimination of offending agents is often incomplete. The syndrome closely resembles the behavioral symptom complex frequently seen in celiac children before they are placed on a gluten-free diet and in infants with milk-induced gastrointestinal bleeding before cow's milk has been withdrawn and iron administered. Undoubtedly, many of the symptoms reflect a chronic hypersensitivity state, perhaps related to excessive release of chemical mediators or lymphokines into the circulation. When iron deficiency anemia is also present, an additional factor causes certain symptoms and intensification of others, often welding the condition into the allergy syndrome. The two causative factors are most readily recognized in such instances by removing the offending allergen and then starting iron therapy one week later. That technique is sometimes impractical when anemia is severe,

Manifestations

but it has been used in some cases by first giving blood transfusions and iron and then eliminating milk a week later. Two distinct stages of improvement have been seen, one sometimes being more striking than the other, depending on the individual circumstances.

URINARY MANIFESTATIONS

The urinary tract is seldom thought of as a potential shock organ for IgE-mediated allergic reactions, although histologically, like the gastrointestinal and respiratory tracts, it has a smooth muscle layer, blood vessels, and mucosa. Judged by the scarcity of reports in the literature, investigators have not adequately considered the possibility of such reactions in the urinary tract. On the other hand, much has been written about kidney involvement in type II hypersensitivity involving antitissue antibodies, e.g., Goodpasture's syndrome. Even more has been written about the role of type III hypersensitivity with immune-complex deposition in renal disease, perhaps the best known and most striking example is that of the renal lesions of disseminated lupus erythematosus. It is beyond the scope of this book to discuss in detail the mechanisms and manifestations of hypersensitivity in urinary tract diseases. One should bear in mind that all four types of allergy may occur, and one should keep an open and observant mind with regard to the possibility of sensitivity to cow's milk affecting different parts of the urinary tract through varying mechanisms. A few provocative observations have already been made.

1. *Enuresis.* Enuresis may result from several causative factors. That allergy is one of the causes of enuresis was suggested in 1931, when Bray[129] noted that when children with asthma avoided the offending allergens, coexisting enuresis sometimes disappeared. In 1959, Breneman[130] described 24 cases of enuresis in which cow's milk, alone, or in association with other foods, was suspected to be a causative allergen. In all patients, the enuresis disappeared after an elimination diet was begun. From his experience, Breneman believed that food allergy was a common cause of nocturnal enuresis, with cow's milk being the leading causative allergen. In another study, the same author[131] subjected 100 children with primary nocturnal enuresis to a dual treatment regimen. Addition of an elimination diet to the bedtime medication increased the cure rate by 26.2 percent. Challenge testing, by feedings of offending foods after symptoms had subsided, provoked enuresis in 53 percent.

Gerrard and co-workers have made additional interesting observations on the role of allergy in enuresis. More enuretic children had allergic disorders than did normal controls.[132] When children with nocturnal enuresis were given a diet free from milk and free from certain other foods, about one-fifth

had an increase in maximum bladder capacity, a fall in diurnal frequency of micturition, and cessation of enuresis.[133, 134] These studies suggest that milk allergy can result in chronic contraction or decreased relaxation of bladder musculature, causing urinary frequency and enuresis.
2. *Cystitis.* In some patients, allergic reactions in the urinary tract may result in symptoms that mimic cystitis, urethritis, or other lesions in the lower genitourinary tract.[120, 135-138] Patients with frequency of micturition, burning, fever, nocturia, urgency, dysuria, hematuria, or urinary retention who did not improve satisfactorily from conventional urologic treatment frequently improved dramatically with appropriate treatment for allergy, including avoidance of allergens, the use of antihistaminics, and in some cases hyposensitization therapy.[138, 141] Some patients with interstitial cystitis had a striking eosinophilic infiltration in the submucosa. Eosinophils in the urine have been noted by some authors[142] but not by others.[138]
3. *Orthostatic albuminuria.* Matsumura and co-workers[143] demonstrated that orthostatic albuminuria could result from hypersensitivity to foods, and even used the appearance of proteinuria after food challenge as a test for food allergy. In 16 cases related to food allergy, cow's milk was an offending allergen in 12.
4. *Nephrotic syndrome.* As has long been known, the nephrotic syndrome is occasionally provoked by bee stings.[144, 145] In some subjects, the nephrotic syndrome is exacerbated during seasonal exposure to specific pollens and hyposensitization may result in remission.[146, 147] In some patients, IgE was demonstrated in the glomerular capillary wall.[148] Groshong and co-workers[149] showed that subjects with nephrotic syndrome had higher levels of serum IgE than patients with other forms of renal disease. Mansfield and colleagues[150] found that serum IgE levels tended to be high in childhood nephrotic syndrome in relapse, whereas IgG levels were low. After successful induction of remission with corticosteroid therapy, the mean serum IgE level declined to normal and the mean IgG rose toward normal. Active hypersensitivity appeared to cause an increased IgE production in most subjects, although the increase was not always reflected in the serum level because of concomitant urinary loss during periods of extreme proteinuria. In a study of more than 100 adult subjects with the nephrotic syndrome, no evidence of an elevated mean serum IgE level was found, nor was there a significant decrease in mean serum IgE after steroid therapy. In this regard, adult-onset nephrotic syndrome appears to differ from childhood-onset syndrome.

In a few selected patients, Matsumura et al.[151] showed that the proteinuria in children with nephrotic syndrome was either induced or aggravated by the ingestion of a specific food; cow's milk was implicated in some subjects. A role of cow's milk allergy in the pathogenesis of the idiopathic nephrotic syndrome was also suggested in a study of six children by Sandberg and co-workers.[152] All six had frequent relapses of nephrotic syndrome that was responsive to repeated courses of steroids. Five of the six had histories of asthma or eczema. Intradermal skin-testing with cow's milk gave positive reactions in all patients. Renal biopsy specimens showed normal structure by light microscopy, and immunofluorescence studies showed no immune-complex deposits in the glomeruli. When cow's milk was replaced by an elemental diet, proteinuria was reduced without corticosteroid therapy. An oral challenge with one ounce of cow's milk resulted in a significant proteinuria, edema, and a decreased urine output. Four patients also had a decrease in serum IgG, and all six patients had an activation of C3. Serum IgA, IgM, and IgE remained within normal range. A remission occurred within 3 to 10 days after withdrawal of cow's milk.

Thus, all clinicians caring for children with the nephrotic syndrome should consider the possibility of food-related exacerbations. Greater use of elimination diets and food challenges are needed. Additional laboratory research into pathogenetic mechanisms and into methods of intervention are also indicated.

CARDIOVASCULAR MANIFESTATIONS

1. *Anaphylactic shock.* Systemic anaphylactic reactions to cow's milk are rare, but an awareness of their occurrence is important. They usually develop rapidly after exposure to cow's milk and may occur after a few drops or milliliters have been ingested.[153,154] The symptoms include sudden weakness; profound pallor; sweating; subnormal temperature; rapid, weak pulse; and hypotension. Frequently associated symptoms are generalized urticaria, angioedema, laryngeal edema, cyanosis, wheezing, abdominal pain, vomiting, diarrhea, or seizures. Subjects who are sensitive to the ingestion of small amounts of cow's milk should be challenged with caution because systemic anaphylaxis may occur, even in patients who previously manifested only mild symptoms of allergy. In milk-sensitive subjects challenged under observation, anaphylaxis was noted in 9 to 33 percent shortly after the ingestion of small quantities of milk.[2,16,59]

Fortunately cow's milk has no use as a parenteral nutrient. In a case report by Wallace et al.,[155] 100 ml of pasteurized cow's milk was inadvertently given by intravenous infusion to a patient with duodenal ulcer. A systemic reaction and urticaria occurred within 10 minutes, followed by disseminated intravascular coagulation and fat embolism. Serum antibodies to milk proteins were not detected by hemagglutination or precipitation tests. The patient showed no adverse reactions to milk feedings 6 weeks later. Whether the immediate reaction in this case was caused by milk proteins or by bacterial antigens in milk is not clear.

2. *Coronary heart disease.* In an epidemiologic study by Briggs and co-workers in 1960,[156] the incidence of myocardial infarction in patients on a high-milk intake was higher than expected. This observation stimulated some investigators to study the immunologic response to cow's milk proteins in patients with coronary heart disease. In a retrospective study of the incidence of coronary artery disease in young persons at autopsy, Osborn[157] noted that in those who were never fed breast milk the coronary arteries were usually abnormal, whereas in those who were breast-fed for 2 months or more the coronary arteries were mostly normal.

In 1969, Davies and co-workers[158] reported an increase in the serum level of hemagglutinating antibodies to cow's milk in coronary heart disease. The elevation of antibodies to constituents in heat-dried milk was considerable, but it was much less for antibodies to constitutents of unheated milk. Because of these observations, Davies postulated that an immunologic mechanism might be involved in atherosclerotic cardiovascular disease.[159-161] He believes that circulating antigen-antibody complexes may be formed in excessive quantities in milk drinkers, and over a period of many years endothelial damage, platelet adherence, plaque formation, and thrombosis may result. A subsequent study[162] suggested that a higher proportion of patients with myocardial infarction than of controls had circulating hemagglutinating antibodies to antigens in milk, and to a lesser extent to antigens in egg. The differences were most striking in patients who died within 6 months of a myocardial infarction.

Studies by other investigators, however, have not supported the hypothesis of an immunologic pathogenesis in coronary heart disease. In two studies,[163, 164] the level of antibodies to milk did not differ between patients with myocardial infarction and age-matched controls. Further studies and more pertinent observations, preferably prospective studies beginning in infancy and accompanied by careful immunologic investigations, are needed to prove or disprove a role for cow's milk allergy in the pathogenesis of coronary heart disease.

3. *Cor pulmonale.* The report[88] on cardiac enlargement and failure of the right side of the heart in three children with high titers of milk precipitins in the serum was referred to earlier. All three had pulmonary hemosiderosis, allergic rhinitis, and hypertrophied adenoids. Each had sleeping hypercapnia and mild respiratory acidosis. The patients clinically improved on a milk-free diet, but complete normalization of the heart size did not occur until adenoidectomy was done.

4. *Cardiac arrhythmias.* The heart as a shock organ of allergy was reported by a number of investigators.[165-168] Cardiac arrhythmias from allergy have been noted more in adults. Rea[169] reported a case of ventricular fibrillation and hypotension in a 68-year-old man who had cardiac shock requiring

resuscitation and vasopressor therapy for 2 days. When the patient was out of shock and off vasopressor therapy, he was offered oral feedings. Immediately after a meal, he developed bloating, had premature ventricular contractions, and his blood pressure dropped. After multiple recurrences, these reactions were found to occur every time he ate milk or eggs.

MISCELLANEOUS MANIFESTATIONS

1. *Failure to thrive.* Poor growth is a frequent finding in children with cow's milk allergy, particularly when the shock organ is the gastrointestinal tract and there is poor appetite, vomiting, diarrhea, malabsorption, exudative enteropathy, or bleeding. In a series of infants with gastrointestinal milk allergy, about one-half had both height and weight below the third percentile.[16] Poor weight gain was also prominent in the patients with chronic pulmonary disease and milk precipitins described by Heiner and co-workers.[83]

2. *Sudden infant death syndrome.* The sudden infant death syndrome (SIDS) or "cot death" is a common diagnosis in infants who die unexpectedly while asleep. Several hypotheses have been proposed to explain the frequent occurrence of SIDS but as yet none has gained wide acceptance or led to a solution of this mysterious malady.

One hypothesis that stimulated much discussion in the literature during the past two decades is that SIDS results from cow's milk anaphylaxis that is modified because it occurs during sleep. The hypothesis is that a sensitized formula-fed infant who is given cow's milk shortly before sleeping regurgitates some stomach contents and aspirates a small amount of the milk into the lungs, where it triggers an acute anaphylactic reaction and sudden death. Such a hypothesis has gained some epidemiologic support from the observation that bottle-fed infants more commonly develop SIDS than breast-fed infants.[170-175] In some reports, however, the feeding pattern of infants with SIDS did not differ from controls.[176-178]

Support for the anaphylaxis hypothesis has also come from immunologic studies both in animal and in man. Parish et al.[170,179] administered small quantities of milk into the larynx of conscious parenterally sensitized guinea pigs, and a typical systemic anaphylactic reaction resulted. The clinical reaction and the pathologic findings, however, differed from those seen in infants with SIDS. But if the guinea pigs were lightly anesthetized, introduction of milk into the larynx invariably resulted in sudden cessation of breathing and death without a struggle; the pathologic findings here resembled those in infants with SIDS. Similar results were noted using orally sensitized animals.[180]

Sera of infants with SIDS have been shown to have antibodies to cow's milk proteins of various immunoglobulin classes, including IgM, IgG, IgA, and IgE.[170, 181, 185] Also, the milk-protein fractions beta-lactoglobulin and alpha-lactalbumin were detected in the lungs and sera of SIDS infants in a higher proportion than in controls.[181] Other investigators, however, have reported similar levels of serum antibodies to cow's milk in SIDS children and in normal children.[186, 189]

The hypothesis of anaphylactic sensitivity to cow's milk in SIDS was not supported when tissue specimens from SIDS infants and from those who died from other recognizable causes were compared by immunofluorescence techniques. Tissues from the two groups showed no significant difference in the number of cells containing antibodies to casein, beta-lactoglobulin, or alpha-lactalbumin.[190] That finding, of course, does not disprove that anaphylaxis is an important cause of SIDS, just as the evidence currently available only suggests that it might be. Although at present there is no convincing evidence for a role of cow's milk allergy in SIDS, the possible beneficial role of breast-feeding should not be forgotten. Immunologically-active constituents of the mother's milk may well serve to augment the newborn's defense mechanisms against foreign proteins during the rather perilous transition from intrauterine life to well-adjusted independent extrauterine life.[174]

3. *Infantile cortical hyperostosis.* The signs and symptoms of infantile cortical hyperostosis, or Caffey's disease, are extreme irritability and deep, tender, soft tissue swellings resembling deep abcesses or osteomyelitis but without regional lymph node enlargement. In early stages, the roentgenogram shows a normal appearance of the bones, but later subperiosteal bone thickening becomes manifest. The mandible, clavicle, and ulna are most frequently affected. The commonly associated laboratory findings are increased erythrocyte sedimentation rate and serum alkaline phosphatase. As a rule, the patient completely recovers within a few months, or in several months, without any treatment. The cause is unknown. An allergic phenomenon was suggested by Bowman et al.,[191] who reported a dramatic improvement in two infants with the disease when they were fed soy formula and a recurrence of symptoms when cow's milk was added to the diet. To our knowledge, this observation has not been substantiated by other studies, and the cause of the disease remains obscure.

4. *Ocular allergy.* A few patients with *allergic conjunctivitis*[120] and *allergic keratitis*[192] from food allergy, including cow's milk, have improved on elimination of the offending food.

5. *Leukorrhea.* Leukorrhea from food allegy has been reported in several women and young girls. In one patient who had facial edema and leukorrhea from milk ingestion, symptoms disappeared after milk was eliminated, and it recurred within a few days after a few drops of diluted milk were added to her diet.[120]

REFERENCES

1. Clein NW: Cow's milk allergy in infants. Pediatr Clin North Am 4:949–962, 1954
2. Goldman AS, Anderson DW, Jr, Sellers WA, et al.: Milk allergy. I. Oral challenge with milk and isolated milk proteins in allergic children. Pediatrics 32:425–443, 1963
3. Gerrard JW, MacKenzie JWA, Goluboff N, et al.: Cow's milk allergy: Prevalence and manifestations in an unselected series of newborns. Acta Paediatr Scand Suppl 234:1–21, 1973
4. Lebenthal E: Cow's milk protein allergy. Pediatr Clin North Am 22:827–833, 1975
5. Davidson M, Burnstine RC, Kugler MM, et al.: Malabsorption defect induced by ingestion of beta lacto-globulin. J Pediatr 66:545–554, 1965
6. Visakorpi JK, Immonen P: Intolerance to cow's milk and wheat gluten in the primary malabsorption syndrome in infancy. Acta Paediatr Scand 56:49–56, 1967
7. Freier S, Kletter B, Gery I, et al.: Intolerance to milk protein. J Pediatr 75:623–631, 1969
8. Lebenthal E, Laor J, Lewitus Z, et al.: Gastrointestinal protein loss in allergy to cow's milk β-lactoglobulin. Israel J Med Sci 6:506–510, 1970
9. Clein NW: Cow's milk allergy in infants and children. Int Arch Allergy 13:245–256, 1958
10. Kuitunen P, Visakorpi JK, Savilahti E, et al.: Malabsorption syndrome with cow's milk intolerance. Arch Dis Child 50:351–356, 1975
11. Freier S, Kletter B: Milk allergy in infants and young children. Clin Pediatr 9:449–454, 1970
12. Freier S, Kletter B: Clinical and immunological aspects of milk protein intolerance. Aust Paediatr J 8:140–146, 1972
13. Matsumura T, Kuroume T, Tajima S: Acetonemic vomiting from viewpoint of food allergy. Acta Allergol (Kbh) 25:423–450, 1970
14. Kane S: Nutritional management of allergic reactions to cow's milk. Am Practit 8:65–69, 1957
15. Wessel MA, Cobb JC, Jackson EB, et al.: Paroxysmal fussing in infancy, sometimes called colic. Pediatrics 14:421–435, 1954
16. Gryboski JD: Gastrointestinal milk allergy in infants. Pediatrics 40:354–362, 1967
17. Brown ET: Proctalgia fugax infantum. Ann Allergy 29:99–100, 1971
18. Speer F: Colic and allergy: A ten year study. Arch Pediatr 75:271–278, 1958
19. Speer F: The allergic tension-fatigue syndrome. Pediatr Clin North Am 1:1029–1037, 1954
20. Deamer WC: Recurrent abdominal pain: A frequent manifestation of food allergy. Curr Med Dialog 40:130–154, 1973
21. Crook WG: Food allergy: The great masquerader. Pediatr Clin North Am 22:227–238, 1975
22. Buisseret PD: Common manifestations of cow's milk allergy in children. Lancet 1:304–305, 1978
23. Liu H-Y, Tsao MU, Moore B, et al.: Bovine milk protein-induced intestinal malabsorption of lactose and fat in infants. Gastroenterology 54:27–34, 1968
24. Shwachman H, Lloyd-Still JD, Khaw KT, et al.: Protracted diarrhea of infancy treated by intravenous alimentation. II. Studies of small intestinal biopsy results. Am J Dis Child 125:365–368, 1973
25. Heiner DC: Gastrointestinal allergy. Prac Pediatr 2:1–16, 1974
26. Morin CL, Buts JP, Weber A, et al: One-hour blood-xylose test in diagnosis of cow's milk allergy. Lancet 2:589, 1976
27. Taylor KB, Thomson DL, Truelove SC, et al.: An immunological study of coeliac disease and idiopathic steatorrhea. Br Med J 2:1727–1731, 1961
28. Sewell P, Cooke WT, Cox EV, et al.: Milk intolerance in gastrointestinal disorders. Lancet 2:1132–1136, 1963
29. Iyngkaran N, Robinson MJ, Prathap K, et al.: Cow's milk protein-sensitive enteropathy: Combined clinical and histological criteria for diagnosis. Arch Dis Child 53:20–26, 1978

30. Liu H-Y, Whitehouse WM, Giday Z: Proximal small bowel transit pattern in patients with malabsorption induced by bovine milk protein ingestion. Pediatr Radiol 115:415–420, 1975
31. Rubin MI: Allergic intestinal bleeding in new born: Clinical syndrome. Am J Med Sci 200:385–390, 1940
32. Wilson JF, Heiner DC, Lahey ME: Studies on iron metabolism. J Pediatr 60:787–800, 1962
33. Wilson JF, Heiner DC, Lahey ME: Milk-induced gastrointestinal bleeding in infants with hypochromic microcytic anemia. JAMA 189:122–126, 1964
34. Wilson JF, Lahey ME, Heiner DC: Studies on iron metabolism. V. Further observations on cow's milk-induced gastrointestinal bleeding in infants with iron-deficiency anemia. J Pediatr 84:335–344, 1974
35. Waldmann TA, Wochner RD, Laster L, et al.: Allergic gastroenteropathy: A cause of excessive gastrointestinal protein loss. N Engl J Med 276:761–769, 1967
36. Santulli TV: Acute necrotizing enterocolitis: Recognition and management. Hosp Pract 11:129–135, 1974
37. Lake AM, Walker WA: Neonatal necrotizing enterocolitis: A disease of altered host defense. Clin Gastroenterol 6:463–480, 1977
38. Aziz EM: Neonatal pneumatosis intestinalis associated with milk intolerance. Am J Dis Child 125:560–562, 1973
39. Powell GK: Enterocolitis in low-birth-weight infants associated with milk and soy protein intolerance. J Pediatr 88:840–844, 1976
40. Powell GK: Milk- and soy-induced entercolitis of infancy: Clinical features and standardization of challenge. J Pediatr 93:553–560, 1978
41. De Peyer E, Walker-Smith J: Cow's milk intolerance presenting as necrotizing enterocolitis. Helv Paediatr Acta 32:509–515, 1977
42. Truelove SC: Ulcerative colitis provoked by milk. Br Med J 1:154–165, 1961
43. Sacca JD: Acute ischemic colitis due to milk allergy. Ann Allergy 29:268–269, 1971
44. Acheson ED, Truelove SC: Early weaning in the etiology of ulcerative colitis: A study of feeding in infancy in cases and controls. Br Med J 2:929–933, 1961
45. Taylor KB, Truelove SC: Circulating antibodies to milk proteins in ulcerative colitis. Br Med J 2:924–929, 1961
46. Davidson L: Milk proteins in ulcerative colitis. Br Med J 2:1358, 1961
47. Dudek B, Spiro HH, Thayer WR: A study of ulcerative colitis and circulating antibodies to milk proteins. Gastroenterology 49:544–547, 1965
48. Mani V, Lloyd G, Green FHY, et al.: Treatment of ulcerative colitis with oral disodium cromoglycate: A double-blind controlled trial. Lancet 1:439–441, 1976
49. Speer F: The allergic child. Am Fam Phys 11:88–94, 1975
50. Speer F: Food allergy: The 10 common offenders. Am Fam Phys 13:106–112, 1976
51. Freier S: Paediatric gastrointestinal allergy. J Hum Nutr 30:187–192, 1976
52. Taub SJ: Food allergies can masquerade as throat cancers. Eye, Ear, Nose & Throat Monthly 48:589–590, 1969
53. Silver H, Douglas DM: Milk intolerance in infancy. Arch Dis Child 43:17–22, 1968
54. Lubos MC, Gerrard JW, Buchan DJ: Disaccharidase activities in milk-sensitive and celiac patients. J Pediatr 10:325–331, 1967
55. Ament ME: Malabsorption syndromes in infancy and childhood. Part I. J Pediatr 81:685–697, 1972
56. Baudon JJ, Fontaine JL, Mougenot JF, et al.: Digestive intolerance to cow's milk proteins in infants: Biological and histological study. Arch Fr Pediatr 32:787–801, 1975
57. Shiner M, Ballard J, Smith ME: The small-intestinal mucosa in cow's milk allergy. Lancet 1:136–140, 1975
58. Fontaine JL, Navarro J: Small intestinal biopsy in cow's milk protein allergy in infancy. Arch Dis Child 50:357–362, 1975

59. Walker-Smith JA: Gastrointestinal allergy. Practitioner 220:562–573, 1978
60. Walker-Smith J, Harrison M, Kilby A, et al.: Cow's milk-sensitive enteropathy. Arch Dis Child 53:375–380, 1978
61. Lebenthal E, Antonowicz I, Shwachman H: Enterokinase and trypsin activities in pancreatic insufficiency and diseases of the small intestine. Gastroenterology 70:508–512, 1976
62. Poley JR, Bhatia M, Welsh JD: Disaccharidase deficiency in infants with cow's milk protein intolerance: Response to treatment. Digestion 17:97–107, 1978
63. Shiner M, Kingston D: The mast cell in gastrointestinal allergic disease. International Symposium on the Mast Cell, Davos, Switzerland, 24–26, April 1979
64. Syme J: Investigation and treatment of multiple intestinal food allergy in childhood. International Symposium on the Mast Cell, Davos, Switzerland, 24–26 April 1979
65. Harrison BM, Walker-Smith JA: Reinvestigation of lactose intolerant children: Lack of correlation between continuing lactose intolerance and small intestinal morphology, disaccharidase activity and lactose tolerance tests. Gut 18:48–52, 1977
66. Savilahti E. Immunochemical study of the malabsorption syndrome with cow's milk intolerance. Gut 14:491–501, 1973
67. Shiner M, Ballard J, Brook CGD, et al.: Intestinal biopsy in the diagnosis of cow's milk protein intolerance without acute symptoms. Lancet 2:1060–1063, 1975
68. Harris MJ, Petts V, Penny R: Cow's milk allergy as a cause of infantile colic:Immunofluorescent studies on jejunal mucosa. Aust Paediatr J 13:276–281, 1977
69. Kilby A, Walker-Smith JA, Wood CBS: Small intestinal mucosa in cow's milk allergy. Lancet 1:531, 1975
70. Bachman KD, Dees SC: Milk allergy. II. Observations on incidence and symptoms of allergy to milk in allergic infants. Pediatrics 20:400–407, 1957
71. Gerrard JW, Lubos MC, Hardy LW, et al.: Milk allergy: Clinical picture and familial incidence. Can Med Assoc J 97:780–785, 1967
72. Endré L, Osvath P: Antigen-induced lymphoblast transformation in the diagnosis of cow's milk allergic diseases in infancy and early childhood. Acta Allergol (Kbh) 30:34–42, 1975
73. Gerrard JW: Familiar recurrent rhinorrhea and bronchitis due to cow's milk. JAMA 198:605–607, 1966
74. Sobien-Kopczynska S, Denys A, Mazur-Cybulska J: Passive hemagglutination test in detection of hypersensitivity to cow's milk in children with recurrent spastic bronchitis and pneumonia. Bull Pol Med Sci Hist 13:120–123, 1970
75. Bahna SL: A statistical study of allergic disorders among school children. Thesis for Doctorate Degree in Public Health, University of Alexandria, Egypt, 1970
76. Sly RM: Exercise related changes in airway obstruction: Frequency and clinical correlates in asthmatic children. Ann Allergy 28:1–16, 1970
77. Heiner DC, Sears JW: Chronic respiratory disease associated with multiple circulating precipitins to cow's milk. Am J Dis Child 100:500–502, 1960
78. Hinkle NH, Hong R, West CD: Identification of the antigen and symptomatology of children with precipitins to milk. Am J Dis Child 102:449–452, 1961
79. Holland NH, Hong R, Davis NC, et al.: Significance of precipitating antibodies to milk proteins in the serum of infants and children. J Pediatr 61:181–195, 1962
80. Chang CH, Wittig HJ: Heiner's syndrome. Radiology 92:507–508, 1969
81. Lee SK, Kniker WT, Cook CD, Heiner DC: Cow's milk induced pulmonary disease in children, in Barness LA (ed): Advances in Pediatrics, vol 25. Chicago, Year Book, 1978, pp 39–57
82. Diner WC, Kniker WT, Heiner DC: Roentgenologic manifestations in the lungs in milk allergy. Radiology 77:564–572, 1961
83. Heiner DC, Sears JW, Kniker WT. Multiple precipitins to cow's milk in chronic respiratory disease. Am J Dis Child 103:634–654, 1962

84. Euler AR, Byrne WJ, Ament ME, et al.: Recurrent pulmonary disease in children: A complication of gastroesophageal reflux. Pediatrics 63:47–51, 1979
85. Soergel KH, Sommers SC: Idiopathic pulmonary hemosiderosis and related syndromes. Am J Med 32:499–511, 1962
86. Heiner DC: Pulmonary hemosiderosis, in Gellis S, Kagan B (eds): Current Pediatric Therapy (ed 5). Philadelphia, Saunders, 1971, pp 139–141
87. Heiner DC: Pulmonary hemosiderosis, in Kendig EL Jr (ed): Disorders of the Respiratory Tract in Children. Philadelphia, Saunders, 1977, pp 538–552
88. Boat TF, Polmar SH, Whitman V, et al.: Hyperreactivity to cow's milk in young children with pulmonary hemosiderosis and cor pulmonale secondary to nasopharyngeal obstruction. J Pediatr 87:23–29, 1975
89. Stafford HA, Polmar SH, Boat TF: Immunologic studies in cow's milk-induced pulmonary hemosiderosis. Pediatr Res 11:898–903, 1977
90. Heiner DC, Rose B: Elevated levels of IgE (γE) in conditions other than classical atopy. J Allergy 45:30–42, 1970
91. Cochrane CG: Mechanisms involved in the deposition of immune complexes in tissues. J Exp Med 134:Suppl 75–89, 1971
92. Brentjens JR, O'Connell DW, Powlowski IB, et al.: Experimental immune complex disease of the lung, the pathogenesis of a laboratory model resembling certain human interstitial lung disease. J Exp Med 140:105–125, 1974
93. Bevenniste J, Egido J, Gutiarrez-Millet V: Evidence for the involvement of the IgE-basophil system in acute serum sickness. Clin Exp Immunol 26:449–456, 1976
94. McGovern JP, Haywood TJ, Fernandez AA: Allergy and serous otitis media. JAMA 200:124–128, 1967
95. Arbesman CE, Ishikawa T, Kroyanek D, et al.: Demonstration of IgA piece in secretions from patients with serous otitis. J Allergy Clin Immunol 49:134, 1972
96. Reisman RE, Bernstein J: Allergy and secretory otitis media. Pediatr Clin North Am 22:251–257, 1975
97. Dees SC, Lefkowitz D III: Secretory otitis media in allergic children. Am J Dis Child 124:364–368, 1972
98. Bland RD: Otitis media, milk allergy, and folk medicine. Pediatrics 50:346, 1972
99. Rapp DJ, Fahey DJ: Allergy and chronic secretory otitis media. Pediatr Clin North Am 22:259–264, 1975
100. Hammar H: Provocation with cow's milk and cereals in atopic dermatitis. Acta Derm Venereol (Stockh) 57:159–163, 1977
101. Eppig JJ: Seborrhea capitis in infants: A clinical experience in therapy. Ann Allergy 29:323–324, 1971
102. Golbert TM, Patterson R, Pruzansky JJ: Systemic allergic reactions to ingested antigens. J Allergy 44:96–107, 1969
103. Matthews TS, Soothill JF: Complement activation after milk feeding in children with cow's milk allergy. Lancet 2:893–895, 1970
104. Whitfield MF, Barr DGD: Cow's milk allergy in the syndrome of thrombocytopenia with absent radius. Arch Dis Child 51:337–343, 1976
105. Jones RHT: Congenital thrombocytopenia and milk allergy. Arch Dis Child 52:744–745, 1977
106. Pock-Steen OC, Niordson A-M: Milk sensitivity in dermatitis herpetiformis. Br J Dermatol 83:614–619, 1970
107. Kuitunen P, Visakorpi JK, Hallman N: Histopathology of duodenal mucosa in malabsorption syndrome induced by cow's milk. Ann Paediatr 205:54–63, 1965
107a. Schur S, Russell A: Milk sensitivity and total alopecia. X International Congress of Allergology, Jerusalem, November 4-11, 1979, p 285

108. Heiner DC, Wilson JF, Lahey ME: Sensitivity to cow's milk. JAMA 189:563–567, 1964
109. Woodruff CW, Clark JL: The role of fresh cow's milk in iron deficiency. I. Albumin turnover in infants with iron deficiency anemia. Am J Dis Child 124:18–23, 1972
110. Lambert PH, Salmon J: Reactions antigene-anticorps et coagulation intravasculaire. Acta Allergol (Kbh) 22:209–219, 1967
111. Storck H: Über Testmethoden bei Nahrungsmitt-elallergie. In Arch Allergy Suppl 3:79–90, 1952
112. Storck H, Bigllardi P, Brenn H, et al.: Über die Bedeutung der Thrombocyten bei allergischen Vongängen, Schweiz Med Wochenschr 83:692–697, 1953
113. Osvath P, Markus M: Diagnostic value of thrombopenia and eosinophilia after food ingestion in children with milk and egg allergy. Acta Paediatr Acad Sci Hung 9:279–284, 1968
114. Church JA, Wang DW, Swanson V, et al.: Cow's milk allergy in a premature infant with hypereosinophilia and hyperimmunoglobulinemia E. Ann Allergy 41:307–310, 1978
115. Ottesen EA, Cohen SG: The eosinophil, eosinophilia and eosinophil-related disorders, in Middleton E, Jr, Reed CE, Ellis EF(eds): Allergy Principles and Practice, vol II. St. Louis, The Mosby 1978, pp 584–632
116. Randolph TG: Allergy as a causative factor of fatigue, irritability and behavior problems of children. J Pediatr 31:560–572, 1947
117. Clarke TW: The part of allergy in childhood neuroses. J Child Psychiatry 1:177–180, 1948
118. Davison HM: Allergy of the nervous system. Quart Rev Allergy 6:157–188, 1952
119. Speer F: Allergy of the Nervous System. Springfield, Ill., Thomas, 1970
120. Rowe AH; Food Allergy: Its Manifestations and Control, and the Elimination Diets: A Compendium. Springfield, Thomas, 1972, pp 334–431
121. Campbell MB: Neurologic manifestations of allergic disease. Ann Allergy 31:485–498, 1973
122. Campbell MB: Neurological and psychiatric aspects of allergy. Otolaryngol Clin North Am 7:805–825, 1974
123. Hilsinger RL: Allergic headaches. Otolaryngol Clin North Am 7:789–803, 1974
124. Tryphonas H, Trites R: Food allergy in children with hyperactivity, learning disabilities and/or minimal brain dysfunction. Ann Allergy 42:22–27, 1979
125. Baldwin DG, Kittler FJ, Ramsay RC Jr: The relationship of allergy to cerebral dysfunction. South Med J 61:1039–1041, 1968
126. Crook WG, Harrison WW, Crawford SE, et al.: Systemic manifestations due to allergy: Report of fifty patients and a review of the literature on the subject (allergic toxemia and the allergic tension-fatigue syndrome). Pediatrics 27:790–799, 1961
127. Weinberg EG, Tuchinda M: Allergic tension-fatigue syndrome. Ann Allergy 31:209–211, 1973
128. Crook WG: Letter to the editor. Ann Allergy 34:130–131, 1975
129. Bray GW: Enuresis of allergic origin. Arch Dis Child 6:251–253, 1931
130. Breneman JC: Allergic cystitis: The cause of nocturnal enuresis. GP 20:85–98, 1959
131. Breneman JC: Nocturnal enuresis: A treatment regimen for general use. Ann Allergy 23: 185–191, 1965
132. Zaleski A, Shokier MK, Gerrard JW: Enuresis: Familial incidence and relationship to allergic disorders. Can Med Assoc J 106:30–31, 1972
133. Esperanca M, Gerrard JW: Nocturnal enuresis: Comparison of the effect of imipramine and dietary restrictions on bladder capacity. Can Med Assoc J 101:721–724, 1969
134. Gerrard JW, Zaleski A: Functional bladder capacities in children with enuresis and recurrent urinary infections, in Dickey LD (ed): Clinical Ecology, Springfield, Ill., Thomas, 1976, pp 224–232
135. Eisenstaedt JS: Allergy and drug hypersensitivity of the urinary tract. J Urol 65:154–159, 1951
136. Powell NB, Powell EB: Vesical allergy in females. South Med J 47:841–848, 1954

137. Powell NB: Allergies of the genito-urinary tract. Ann Allergy 19:1019–1025, 1961
138. Powell NB, Powell EB, Thomas OC, et al.: Allergy of the lower urinary tract. J Urol 107:631–634, 1972
139. Powell NB, Boggs PB, McGovern JP: Allergy of the lower urinary tract. Ann Allergy 28:252–255, 1970
140. Horesh AJ: Allergy and recurrent urinary tract infections in childhood. I. Ann Allergy 36:16–22, 1976
141. Horesch AJ: Allergy and recurrent urinary tract infections in childhood. II. Ann Allergy 36:174–179, 1976
142. Pastinszky I: The allergic diseases of the male genitourinary tract with special reference to allergic urethritis and cystitis. Urol Int 9:288–305, 1959
143. Matsumura T, Kuroume T, Fukushima I: Significance of food allergy in the etiology of orthostatic albuminuria. J Asthma Res 3:325–329, 1966
144. Rytand DA: Onset of the nephrotic syndrome during a reaction to bee sting. Stanford Med Bull 3:224–233, 1955
145. Venters HD, Vernier RL, Worthen HC, et al.: Bee sting nephrosis: A study of the immunopathologic mechanisms. Am J Dis Child 102:688–689, 1961
146. Wittig HJ, Goldman AS: Nephrotic syndrome associated with inhaled allergens. Lancet 1:542–543, 1970
147. Reeves WG, Cameron JS, Johansson SGO, et al.: Seasonal nephrotic syndrome: Description and immunological findings. Clin Allergy 5:121–137, 1975
148. Gerber MA, Paronetto F: IgE in glomeruli of patients with nephrotic syndrome. Lancet 1:1097–1099, 1971
149. Groshong T, Mendelson L, Mendoza S, et al.: Serum IgE in patients with minimal-change nephrotic syndrome. J Pediatr 83:767–771, 1973
150. Mansfield LE, Trygstad EW, Ajugwo RE, et al.: Serum levels of IgE, IgG, and alpha 2M in childhood renal disease. J Allergy Clin Immunol 57:230, 1976
151. Matsumura T, Kuroume T, Matsui A, et al.: Therapy of the nephrotic syndrome by eradication of foci and elimination diets. Proceedings of the XIII International Congress of Pediatrics, 1971, pp 41–56
152. Sandberg DH, McIntosh RM, Bernstein CW, et al.: Severe steroid-responsive nephrosis associated with hypersensitivity. Lancet 1:388–390, 1977
153. Park EA: A case of hypersensitiveness to cow's milk. Am J Dis Child 19:46–54, 1920
154. Hill LW: Some advances in pediatric allergy in the last ten years. Pediatr Clin North Am 11:17–31, 1964
155. Wallace JR, Payne RW, Mack AJ: Inadvertent intravenous infusion of milk. Lancet 6:1264–1266, 1972
156. Briggs RD, Rubenberg ML, O'Neal RM, et al.: Myocardial infarction in patients treated with Sippy and other high-milk diets. Circulation 21:538–542, 1960
157. Osborn GR: Stages in development of coronary disease observed from 1,500 young subjects: Relationship of hypotension and infant feeding to etiology. Colloques Int Cent Natn Rech Scient 169:94–139, 1968
158. Davies DF, Davies JR, Richards MA: Antibodies to reconstituted dried cow's milk protein in coronary heart disease. J Atheroscler Res 9:103–107, 1969
159. Davies DF: An immunological view of atherogenesis. J Atheroscler Res 10:253–259, 1969
160. Davies DF: Milk protein and other food antigens in atheroma and coronary heart disease. Am Heart J 81:289–290, 1971
161. Davies DF: Immunological aspects of atherosclerosis. Proc Nutr Soc 35:293–295, 1976
162. Davies DF, Johnson AP, Rees BWG, et al.: Food antibodies and myocardial infarction. Lancet 1:1012–1014, 1974

163. Toivanen A, Viljanen MK, Savilahti E: IgM and IgG anti-milk antibodies measured by radioimmunoassay in myocardial infarction. Lancet 2:205–207, 1975
164. Scott BB, Swinburne ML, McGuffin P, et al.: Dietary antibodies and myocardial infarction. Lancet 2:125–126, 1976
165. Bernstein C, Klotz SD: Allergy and the heart in clinical practice. Ann Allergy 8:336–344, 1950
166. Harkavy J: Cardiac manifestations due to hypersensitivity. Ann Allergy 28:242–251, 1970
167. Boxer RW: Cardiac arrythmias due to foods, in Dickey LD (ed): Clinical Ecology. Springfield, Ill, Thomas, 1976, pp 193–200
168. Klotz SD: Allergy and the cardiovascular system, in Dickey LD (ed): Clinical Ecology. Springfield, Ill., Thomas, 1976, pp 184–192
169. Rea WJ: Environmentally triggered cardiac disease. Ann Allergy 40:243–251, 1978
170. Parish WE, Barrett AM, Coombs RRA, et al.: Hypersensitivity to milk and sudden death in infancy. Lancet 2:1106–1110, 1960
171. Carpenter RG, Shaddick CW: Role of infection, suffocation, and bottle-feeding in cot death: An analysis of 110 cases and their controls. Br J Prev Soc Med 19:1–7, 1965
172. Steele R, Krause AS, Langworth JT: Sudden unexpected death in infancy in Ontario: Part I. Methodology and findings related to the host. Can J Public Health 58:359–364, 1967
173. Frankland AW: Food allergies. R Soc Health J 90:243–247, 1970
174. Gunther M: The neonate's immunity gap, breast feeding, and cot death. Lancet 1:441–442, 1975
175. Biering-Sorensen F, Jorgensen T, Hilden J: Sudden infant death in Copenhagen 1956–1971. I. Infant feeding. Acta Paediatr Scand 67:129–137, 1978
176. Froggatt P, Lynas MA, MacKenzie G: Epidemiology of sudden unexpected death in infants ("cot death") in Northern Ireland. Br J Prev Soc Med 25:119–134, 1971
177. Bergman AB, Ray CG, Pomeroy MA, et al.: Studies of the sudden infant death syndrome in King County, Washington. III. Epidemiology. Pediatrics 49:860–870, 1972
178. Tonkin S: Sudden infant death syndrome: Hypothesis of causation. Pediatrics 55:650–661, 1975
179. Parish WE, Barrett AM, Coombs RRA: Inhalation of cow's milk by sensitized guinea-pigs in the conscious and anaesthetized state. Immunology 3:307–324, 1960
180. Devey ME, Anderson KJ, Coombs RRA, et al.: The modified anaphylaxis hypothesis for cot death: Anaphylactic sensitization in guineapigs fed cow's milk. Clin Exp Immunol 26:542–548, 1976
181. Parish WE, Richards CB, France NE, et al.: Further investigations on the hypothesis that some cases of cot-death are due to a modified anaphylactic reaction to cow's milk. Int Arch Allergy 24:215–243, 1964
182. Hunter A, Feinstein A, Coombs RRA: Immunoglobulin class of antibodies to cow's milk casein in infant sera and evidence for low molecular weight IgM antibodies. Immunology 15:381–388, 1968
183. Parish WE: Detection of reaginic and short-term sensitizing anaphylactic or anaphylactoid antibodies to milk in sera of allergic and normal persons. Clin Allergy 1:369–380, 1971
184. Turner KJ, Baldo BA, Carter RF, et al.: Sudden infant death syndrome in South Australia: Measurement of serum IgE antibodies to three common allergens. Med J Aust 2:855–859, 1975
185. Turner KJ, Baldo BA, Hilton JMN: RAST studies: IgE antibodies to *Dermatogoides pteronyssinus* (house dust mite), *Aspergillus fumigatus* and β-lactoglobulin in sudden death in infancy syndrome (SIDS). Dev Biol Stand 29:208–216, 1975
186. Gold E, Godek G: Antibodies to milk in serum of normal infants and infants who died suddenly and unexpectedly. Am J Dis Child 102:542, 1961

187. Peterson RDA: Antibodies to cow's milk proteins: Their presence and significance. Pediatrics 31:209–221, 1963
188. Johnstone JM, Lawy HS: Role of infection in cot deaths. Br Med J 1:706–709, 1966
189. Clark JW, Yuninger JW, Bonnes PA, et al.: Serum IgE antibodies in sudden infant death syndrome. J Pediatr 95:85–86, 1979
190. Valdes-Dapena MA, Felipe RP: Immunofluorescent studies in crib deaths: Absence of evidence of hypersensitivity to cow's milk. Am J Clin Pathol 56:412–415, 1971
191. Bowman JR, Crosby LF, Jr, Piston RE: Observations on the etiology and therapy of infantile cortical hyperostosis. J Tenn Med Assoc 48:257–260, 1955
192. Ruedemann AD: Ocular allergy. Ohio State Med J 30:304–306, 1934

6
Diagnosis

At the present time, the diagnosis of cow's milk allergy in most instances depends more on clinical evaluation than on laboratory data. The diagnosis is suggested by the clinical history, by symptoms and signs that are known to be caused by milk allergy, and by the exclusion of other conditions that might cause similar manifestations. Verification of the diagnosis should be based on the documentation of an improvement in symptoms after milk has been strictly avoided, a recurrence of symptoms on challenge with milk, and clearing again on a second trial of milk elimination. That documentation is the minimum acceptable three-step requirement for diagnosis. Laboratory tests are of help when done in competent laboratories and interpreted by experienced workers; however, alone, they can seldom prove or exclude the diagnosis. They are most useful when carried out in association with milk elimination and challenge tests. In fact, in such circumstances, altered measurements of physiologic, biochemical, or histologic activity responding to elimination and challenge tests constitute the most reliable evidence currently available to confirm the diagnosis of allergy to cow's milk or other foods.

Because more than one immunologic mechanism is involved in the pathogenesis of milk allergy, no single immunologic procedure can be depended upon to support the diagnosis in all cases. Maximal benefit from laboratory tests requires an intellectual choice of critical tests in the light of the clinical picture and acknowledge of the most likely underlying immunologic mechanism (see Chap. 4). As must be kept in mind, more immunologic reactions than one are often involved in the pathogenesis of symptoms in any particular patient.

The need for caution in diagnosing allergy to cow's milk can hardly be overemphasized. Overzealous diagnoses may result both in missing the real cause of the patient's symptoms and in unnecessarily restricting the use of milk and milk-containing foods. A general outline for diagnostic procedures of milk allergy is presented below:

> Suggestive
> > History of association between symptoms and milk ingestion
> > Family history of allergy, especially to cow's milk
> > Clinical manifestations, absence of causes other than allergy
>
> Verification
> > Milk elimination-challenge test
>
> Auxiliary aids
> > Skin-testing: epicutaneous; intracutaneous; contact; skin window; passive transfer
> > Eosinophilia: blood; local secretion
> > Serum immunoglobulins, including total IgE
> > Specific antibodies to milk proteins: RAST; ELISA; precipitation; hemagglutination; complement-fixation; immune-complexes
> > In vitro tests on leukocytes: leukocyte histamine release; cytotoxic food test; lymphoblast transformation; lymphokine production
> > Intestinal mucosal biopsy

HISTORY AND CLINICAL PICTURE

The first and most valuable clues of allergy to cow's milk are often derived from a careful history. There one finds the first clue to the allergic nature of a patient's symptoms and the first indication of the allergens to be suspected. The history should include inquiry into the mode of feeding, dietary habits, nature of symptoms and age of onset, and a detailed evaluation of the circumstances existing at or just before the appearance of symptoms. Cow's milk allergy is more prevalent in young children than in older age groups. It is more common children who were bottle-fed from birth than in those who were initially breast-fed. Often the child is brought to a physician because of a gastrointestinal, respiratory, or skin problem that started in the neonatal period shortly after formula-feeding was begun or when homogenized cow's milk was introduced into the diet. Milk allergy should be considered in infants who have unexplained iron deficiency anemia, or in children of any age with chronic or recurrent pulmonary disease. It should be considered as a possible cause of thrombocytopenia, behavior disorders, and a wide variety of subjective complaints. A past or current history of other allergies increases the likelihood that an immunologic mechanism underlies the symptoms.

An association between the child's symptoms and ingestion of cow's milk is often unsuspected by the parents, particularly during the first visit. Such an association may be easier to discover in older children or adults if they drink milk infrequently. Even so, symptoms with delayed onset are seldom thought by the patient to bear a relationship to a food that may have been ingested 8 to 24 hours earlier. Cow's milk obviously would be the major suspected food allergen in a young infant whose diet consisted solely or predominantly of a milk formula.

The quantities of milk or milk products ingested by the patient should be cautiously evaluated. In an exquisitely milk-sensitive subject, the ingestion of even minute quantities of milk may result in severe symptoms, whereas in another subject, symptoms may appear only after the intake of large quantities. Although the refusal of a certain food by some children may be a sign of allergy to that food,[1,2] other children may tend to overindulge in the offending food allergen. Randolph[3] referred to this phenomenon as "food addiction," but we prefer the terms *excessive appetite* or *craving* for the food.

The food diary, a frequently used diagnostic aid, is sometimes helpful in cases of hypersensitivity to multiple food items and in those of delayed-onset food allergy reactions. It is of most value when the offending food is not ingested in similar amounts every day. The daily recording of symptoms and of foods ingested over a few weeks can be as rewarding in excluding suspected foods from consideration as in pinpointing the specific offenders. It is of greatest use by experienced investigators who are cautious in its interpretation. The time of occurrence or exacerbation of symptoms, as well as the time and quantity of foods ingested, should be recorded. Patients with infrequent symptoms may be asked to keep a modified food diary in which they record foods taken and possible precipitating events that occurred during the 24 to 72 hours preceding the onset of symptoms.

Family History

A history of allergy in the parents or siblings increases the likelihood that the patient is allergy-prone and that some or all of his symptoms may be manifestations of allergy.

We have observed, as have others,[4-7] a familial tendency to cow's milk intolerance. Deamer[8] noted intolerance to cow's milk in four generations of one family. Gerrard[9] estimated that within any family having one child with milk allergy, a subsequently born sibling will have a 1:3 chance of having problems when fed cow's milk. Coe and Mansmann[10] reported identical twins with cow's milk allergy; both infants had the same manifestations and had positive immediate skin reactions to alpha-lactalbumin, beta-lactoglobulin, and alpha-casein, but not to bovine serum albumin. In some instances in which both a child and a parent had precipitating antibodies to antigens in cow's milk, the precipitins were directed to the same milk constituent(s). That similarity was believed to occur more frequently than when precipitating antibodies of a child were compared with those of unselected adults.[11] Heredity probably plays an important role in determining specific sensitizations.

Clinical Picture

Physical examination is essential not only in properly assessing the extent and nature of a patient's allergy, but also in excluding causes other than allergy for the symptoms. Selected laboratory tests or roentgenologic examinations may also be required. In the presence of suspected milk allergy, the institution of a milk-free diet need not be delayed until all necessary investigations have been completed. On the contrary, a trial on a milk-free diet at an early and appropriate time after the diagnosis has been seriously considered will often obviate the need for costly investigations and unpleasant procedures. Only a carefully conducted challenge feeding may be needed to confirm the diagnosis.

CHALLENGE TESTS

Oral Challenge

As previously mentioned, the most universally applicable diagnostic procedure is the institution of a milk-free diet accompanied by careful observations or physiologic measurements to document clearing or improvement of symptoms and signs, their recurrence by reintroducing the food into the diet, and a second improvement on reeliminating milk from the diet.

Our procedure of oral milk challenge is illustrated in Figure 6-1. When cow's milk allergy is suspected, cow's milk and its products are strictly eliminated for 4 weeks. If the patient has intermittent symptoms or signs similar to those frequently encountered in milk-related pulmonary disease, the milk-free diet must be continued a month longer than the longest symptom-free interval while ingesting milk. Milk-free diets are always more readily achieved in young infants than in older children since infants can be easily fed solely on a cow's milk-substitute such as soybean formula. After the patient has been asymptomatic for 1 to 4 weeks while not taking medications, he is subjected to the challenge test, which should be done under supervision, usually in a hospital or in an outpatient clinic with facilities available to manage any untoward reaction that might occur. One should have epinephrine, intravenous and oral antihistamines, aminophylline, vasopressor agents, intravenous fluids, oxygen, airways, and other emergency provisions available. These precautions are particularly needed when prior reactions to milk have been severe or have occurred after the ingestion of only small amounts (less than 2 ounces) of milk. After a milk-sensitive subject has been strictly avoiding milk for more than a week, the subsequent reaction is often more severe than the initial milk-related symptoms.[12] Shock after challenge has

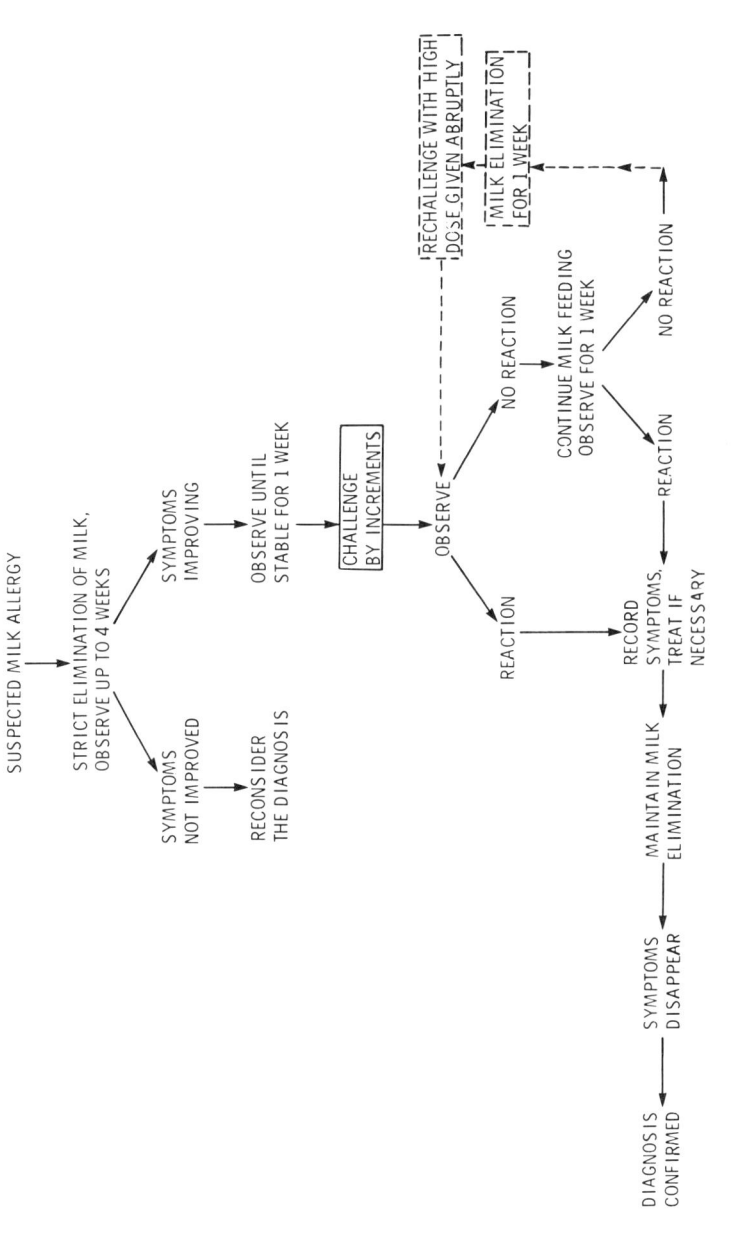

Fig. 6-1. Procedure of oral milk challenge.

been reported in some instances.[13,15] Most such reactions occur in subjects whose parents, or they themselves, are aware of the relationship of milk ingestion to severe symptoms. Such reactions are rare in subjects who have chronic rhinitis, pulmonary disease, or occult gastrointestinal bleeding that results from drinking a liter or more of milk daily. Obviously, if a severe reaction has occurred in the past, the challenge should not be carried out, except under certain circumstances and with great caution.

A prechallenge physical examination must be done, and if the patient has symptoms or signs of allergy, infection, or other illness, the challenge should be postponed. During challenge, the patient should be in a reassuring, relaxed environment, without apprehension from the parents or the person conducting the challenge. In one study,[13] the time of onset of milk-induced symptoms after oral challenge was less than 1 hour in 39 percent, 1 to 5 hours in 21 percent, 6 to 11 hours in 10 percent, 12 to 24 hours in 17 percent, 1 to 3 days in 11 percent, and 7 days in 1 percent.

A suitable milk preparation is either homogenized cow's milk containing 2 percent fat or the cow's milk formula that was thought to cause the patient's symptoms. The dose depends on the quantities previously ingested by the patient and the severity of the symptoms. A child with severe symptoms can first be tested with 1 drop of a 1:100 dilution. At hourly intervals, he can be given 1 drop of 1:10 dilution, 1 drop full strength, 10 drops full strength, 10 ml, and then 100 ml if symptoms have not yet appeared. Children with less severe allergies can begin with 1 drop or 1 ml full strength. In all children, the maximum dose to be given can be reached within 6 to 7 hours in the absence of provocation of serious symptoms. In some children, full feedings may need to be continued for several days to determine the effect of the challenges. The patient should be watched carefully after the ingestion of the test doses. If symptoms or signs of an allergic reaction develop, they should be documented by the best method available, such as description, measurement of pulmonary function or intestinal blood loss, jejunal biopsy, or other pertinent tests. Whenever possible, reactions should be observed by the physician directing the challenge tests. Notes should be carefully recorded before giving the next higher dose until several full doses have been given. If no symptoms or signs develop after the patient has had a generous daily intake for 1 to 2 weeks, the test result is considered negative. Recurrence of symptoms or signs more than doubles the diagnostic credibility of an apparently successful initial elimination diet. The test result, however, is not considered positive before a second disappearance of symptoms and signs has been documented on the reinstitution of a milk-free diet. If the results of the first challenge test are equivocal, a second challenge may be needed in which larger amounts are given more abruptly. We no longer believe it necessary to document three positive challenges, as once advocated.[13] Although symptoms resulting from a positive challenge are usually similar to the original presenting symptoms, they need not be exactly the same. Thus, an infant with low-grade milk-induced occult gastrointestinal bleeding of perhaps 5 ml per day may have no apparent bowel disturbance before being studied. After 5 to 7 days of a milk-free diet with cessation of intestinal blood loss, reintroduction of cow's milk rather commonly provokes not only a recurrence of occult bleeding but also diarrheal stools, colic, or fretful, dependent behavior. No new food other than the milk substitute should be introduced to the basic diet until the diagnosis has been settled.

If it is important to eliminate rigorously the possibility of false-positive reactions or placebo effects, the challenge test must be done double-blind, using the allergen and a placebo on different test occasions without the awareness of the tested subject, or of those doing the test. Double-blind tests are seldom used during infancy, because placebo effects are uncommon in infants under 1 year old, and they are not more universally used in diagnosing food allergy because they are somewhat cumbersome. The use of opaque capsules to contain powdered milk or a placebo[16,17] can be helpful in patients whose symptoms are provoked by quantities of milk that can be contained in a few capsules. Loveless[18] used an antacid emulsion mixed with milk on one occasion and with water as a placebo. The patient was asked to close his eyes and his nostrils until the test meal was brought to him and swallowed. A small nasogastric tube can be inserted through which several hundred milliliters of cow's milk or placebo (soy milk or other suitable substitute) can be introduced in double-blind fashion. In principle, symptoms and signs induced by known milk challenge should be induced by double-blind milk administration but not by placebo. Unfortunately, as experienced investigators are aware, a placebo effect is quite common in food allergic subjects, and can be sorted out only by carefully conducted double-blind studies.

Challenging with individual milk protein fractions has found limited use in clinical practice, since such fractions are not readily available in purified form. Some patients are sensitive solely to heat-labile constituents of cow's milk, such as bovine serum albumin and bovine gamma globulin, and might tolerate heat-treated milk. Such patients can be identified by comparing the effects of challenge with pasteurized homogenized milk to challenge with the same milk brought to a boil. Canned evaporated milk is also a suitable "heat-denatured" milk.

Sublingual Provocation

Provocation testing by the sublingual application of drop quantities of suspected food allergen extracts has been advocated.[19,20] Positive responses are expected to reproduce the patient's symptoms usually within 10 minutes, rarely later.

The Food Allergy Committee of the American College of Allergists evaluated the test on two occasions.[21] Double-blind cross-over studies were carried out on patients with known food allergies. Positive responses to food allergen extracts were similar to those induced by placebo, and the results were similar whether 1:40 or 1:10 weight per volume extracts were used. In our opinion, this study, which was done carefully by competent practicing physicians, underscored the importance of recognizing the frequency and variability of placebo effects.

Subcutaneous Provocation

Rinkel et al.[22] advocated testing for food allergy by provoking symptoms through subcutaneously injecting suspected allergen extracts. The Committee on Provocative Food Testing of the American College of Allergists evaluated the test.[23] Patients with convincing histories of food allergy that had been verified by oral challenge were subjected to double-blind studies in which 0.1 ml of placebo or food extract, 1:100 weight per volume, were subcutaneously injected. Positive responses to most food extracts occurred in the same frequency as to the placebo. Also reproducibility of the results was poor. A study by the Food Committee of the American Academy of Allergy reported similar findings.[24] The conclusion is inescapable that although the subcutaneous injection of food allergen extracts undoubtedly affects some subjects, a significant number of the reactions are actually placebo effects. Placebo effect can be separated from antigen-specific effects only through challenge tests by double-blind protocol.

SKIN-TESTING

Skin-testing is still the most frequently used diagnostic procedure in allergy practice. Several methods are used, but the most popular are the epicutaneous (scratch or prick) and intracutaneous techniques. Unfortunately, both false-positive and false-negative responses to food antigens are frequent.[13, 17, 25-28]

Epicutaneous and Intracutaneous Tests

The epicutaneous (scratch or prick) technique, which minimizes the occurrence of severe reactions, is usually used first, and if the reaction is negative, the investigator often resorts to the intracutaneous technique before pronouncing the entire result negative. For practical purposes, crude extracts or dilutions of skim milk rather than of individual milk protein fractions are usually used. For scratch- or prick-testing, glycerinated extracts are usually used in a concentration of 1:20 or 1:10 weight per volume, whereas for intradermal testing aqueous dilutions of 1:10,000 to 1:100 are preferred, 1:1000 being used most often.[16, 27, 29-31] Control tests should always be included, using the diluent or extracting solution in which the milk proteins are dissolved. Erythema and wheal formation that occur within 15 to 20 minutes suggest type I (immediate) hypersensitivity reactions mediated by IgE, whereas if the formation of erythema and wheal occur 4 to 8 hours later, this suggests an Arthus-like reaction. A skin response after 24 to 72 hours suggests a cell-mediated reaction. For reasons that are not entirely clear, intracutaneous skin tests results are sometimes positive when scratch- or prick-

Diagnosis

test results are negative, even when much greater concentrations of the extract are used in the latter. One can speculate that a different type of antibody such as a heat-stable short-term IgG antibody, perhaps of the IgG4 subclass, might predominate in such responses, but convincing proof has not yet been forthcoming.

The high rate of unreliable responses in skin-testing with food antigens in general can be attributed to several factors, including the following:

1. The antigen preparation may be of poor quality. Preparations from different manufacturers differ widely in potency. Also antigenicity, particularly of whole or fractionated milk proteins, is frequently lost during storage, necessitating the frequent preparation of fresh testing solutions. Greater attention to the potential value of stabilizing agents[32] in preparing food allergens for skin-testing is certainly overdue.
2. False-positive responses are especially frequent in patients with dermographism or dermatoses, in whom the skin reactivity is increased, whereas false-negative responses may be encountered in persons with thickened skin and in old age.
3. The skin response does not necessarily reflect the reactivity of other shock organs. It is common to obtain a positive skin response to an antigen that in natural exposure does not cause symptoms in the patient. Also, undoubted allergy to cow's milk may occur in spite of negative results to skin tests as, for example, in cow's milk-related diarrhea in infants.
4. The routine checking of skin responses once at 15 to 20 minutes overlooks responses that occur after 4 to 8 hours or after 24 to 48 hours. Late responses, though not commonly found, may be of special significance in some instances of cow's milk-related gastrointestinal or pulmonary disease.
5. Patients showing a negative response to whole cow's milk extract occasionally respond positively to purified milk protein fractions, to extracts heated with lactose, or to enzymatic digests of cow's milk protein.[33-35]
6. Either false-negative or false-positive responses may result from poor technique in performing the test, or failure to include proper controls.

Contact Skin Test

Contact skin-testing helps to verify contact allergy to milk.[36] One drop of whole cow's milk, undiluted or diluted 1:20 in normal saline solution, is applied to clean, unscarified skin and inspected for erythema and wheal formation at 15 to 20 minutes. It is then covered by a simple bandage and again inspected at about 6 hours and at 24 to 48 hours.

Skin Window

The skin-window technique was originally devised by Rebuck and Crowley in 1955[37] for the in vivo study of leukocyte migration. Bullock and Bodenbender[29] applied the technique to the diagnosis of food allergy. The skin of the anterior surface of the forearm or of the thigh is scrubbed with an antiseptic solution and dried with a sterile gauze sponge. Small windows about 5 mm in diameter are created by scraping the epidermis with a blade. One drop of skimmed milk, full strength or diluted 1:10 in normal saline solution, is applied on the abraded area and covered with a glass slide that is kept in place for 24 hours. The slide is then stained and examined for eosinophils and other leukocytes. The test result is considered positive if the percentage of eosinophils is 3-fold or more greater than the percentage recovered from a control window where no antigen was applied.

Skin-window responses were frequently positive in immediate-type hypersensitivity reactions but not in delayed allergic reactions.[28,29] In some patients, the test result was negative, although evidence from both history and intradermal tests was positive. Because of its cumbersome nature and limited utility, the skin-window technique is not recommended for routine allergy testing.

Prausnitz-Küstner Passive Transfer Test

The passive transfer test, or Prausnitz-Küstner (P-K) reaction, once served a useful role in demonstrating specific serum reagins. It could be substituted for direct skin-testing in patients with generalized dermatoses or severe dermographism. It was also a valuable research procedure, opening the way for the discovery of IgE by Ishizaka et al.[38] and the development of radioimmunoassay of IgE antibody.[39] The P-K test is now seldom resorted to because of the risk of transmitting viral hepatitis or syphilis. Fortunately, current need for the test has been minimized by the availability of reliable in vitro tests for serum IgE antibodies.

In the P-K test, the patient's serum is collected under aseptic conditions, and it is ascertained to be negative for hepatitis B antigen and for evidence of syphilis. A healthy nonallergic recipient is injected intradermally with 0.02 to 0.1 ml of the patient's serum and in another site with a similar amount of control serum, also known to be free of hepatitis virus or spirochetes. The sites are marked with a pen, and 48 hours later both injection sites are challenged by a solution of the allergen under investigation, which could be whole cow's milk, a purified cow's milk protein, or an allergen (antigen) preparation that had been heat-treated, enzymatically digested, or otherwise altered. In a modification of the usual P-K test, termed the *oral-challenge passive-transfer test,* the recipient is offered the suspected food and the sites of passive serum injection are observed for erythema and wheal formation. The latter procedure requires that antigenically active material escapes digestion or denaturation in the intestinal tract and is absorbed into the circulation, where it is delivered to the skin sites. With either procedure, the suitability of different recipients varies. Bazaral et al.[40] suggested that the reliability of P-K tests could be increased by using recipients with normal serum IgE levels. Other factors such as basophil and mast cell sensitivity for histamine release may be important as well. By diluting the serum used for passive sensitization (e.g., 1:10, 1:100, and 1:1000) the relative amount of reaginic IgE antibody present in the donor's serum can be determined. As with other tests for IgE antibody, the finding of a high level of specific antibody to a cow's milk protein suggests, but does not by itself prove, the existence of clinically important allergy to cow's milk. In general, the higher the antibody titer the more likely there will be clinical allergy, but, as an exception, some patients may have demonstrable reaginic antibody without detectable allergy. Equally important is the occasional finding of a low or undetectable level of reaginic antibody in some subjects who have severe immediate hypersensitivity responses, even anaphylactic shock.

IN VITRO TESTS

Eosinophilia

An increase in the circulating eosinophils provides helpful suggestive evidence of allergy. Eosinophilia has been reported in about one-fourth to one-half of milk-sensitive patients.[41-43] A problem in the clinical evaluation of eosinophil counts in peripheral blood has been the wide range in normal healthy persons, varying from 0 to 600/cu mm, the higher counts being found in children rather than in adults.[44] We consider counts of 400/cu mm or more to be elevated. Eosinophilia per se is only suggestive of allergy because it may be present in association with many other illnesses.[44,45]

In patients with milk allergy, the eosinophil count may show a reduction toward normal after milk has been eliminated from the diet or it may show an increase after milk has been ingested.[46-50]

The number of eosinophils may increase at the site of an allergic reaction as evidenced by accumulations in local secretions of the respiratory or gastrointestinal tract. In the vomitus or stools of patients with gastrointestinal milk allergy, eisoinophils are often found in association with mucus.[51,52] In the stools, the presence of Charcot-Leyden crystals may indicate an increased number of eosinophils, many of which may have been destroyed in the bowl lumen.

Serum Immunoglobulins

Determining total immunoglobulin levels in the serum may provide valuable clues in investigating the cause of symptoms suggestive of milk allergy. Low levels of serum immunoglobulins suggest B cell dysfunction as a cause of the patient's symptoms. A selective deficiency of serum IgA is usually associated with a deficiency in secretory IgA, a major protective factor in the gastrointestinal tract.

Serum IgG, IgA, and IgM are easily measured by means of single radial immunodiffusion plates, which are widely available commercially. Special "low-level plates" may be needed to detect the low immunoglobulin levels normally found in the sera of infants and the levels found in bodily secretions at any age. A recent study suggested that the propensity to develop allergy to cow's milk or to other foods is enhanced during transient hypogammaglobulinemia of infancy.[53]

Serum IgE.

The total serum IgE level is probably best determined by double-antibody[54] or paper-disc[55] radioimmunoassays. An elevated serum IgE level is a common finding in patients with immediate-type hypersensitivity. In infancy and early childhood, about one-half of the patients with milk allergy have elevations in the serum level of IgE.[31, 56-58] Obviously, a normal serum IgE does not exclude the diagnosis of milk allergy. Nevertheless, a high level in the absence of evidence for other diseases is highly suggestive.

A high IgE level may be caused by a variety of conditions other than allergy, including parasitic infestations, bronchopulmonary aspergillosis, liver cirrhosis, multiple myeloma, mucocutaneous lymph node syndrome, and the acute mononucleosis syndrome[59-64]

Radioallergosorbent Test (RAST)

RAST is a radioimmunoassay technique originally described by Wide et al.[39] to detect specific IgE antibodies. It can detect serum IgE antibodies to a wide variety of antigens. In the test for IgE antibodies to cow's milk antigens, cynanogen-bromide-activated paper discs coated with whole cow's milk and others coated with individual protein fractions are used. In general, the results are more meaningful when purified than when crude antigens are used. A minor protein constituent of cow's milk may be a major allergen, yet its concentration on the surface of a paper disc coated with crude milk protein may be insufficient to permit assessment of IgE antibodies directed to it. Our experience with patients allergic to milk has been similiar to that of others in that RAST may be negative in a significant number of patients with obvious milk allergy.[30, 65, 66] In a few instances, a serum that has a negative RAST using discs coated with whole milk or purified milk proteins may have a positive result when discs coated with enzymatic digests of the protein are used.[67] The circumstance, however, seems to occur infrequently, and at the present time RAST studies in which milk protein digests are used appear to be of little help to the clinician.

Low serum levels of IgE antibodies to milk proteins are common in nonallergic persons.[66, 68] Therefore, well-designed studies will always include sera from several healthy control subjects who drink cow's milk as well as known positive and neagtive control sera in the same assay. RAST results and immediate responses to skin-testing with cow's milk antigens have been strongly correlated in some studies,[69-71] but only moderately[66] or weakly[72] correlated in others. RAST has several advanatage for both the investigator and the clinician:

No patient discomfort or risk
A small serum sample is sufficient for several tests
Convenient for patient and physician
Lack of inhibition by medications
Accurate comparisons possible between serial sera from the same patient or between samples from different patients
Test characteristics:
    Fairly quantitative and highly precise
    Good reproducibility
    Standardized and stable reagents utilized
    Subject to quality control
Preferable to skin-testing in:
    Infants and young children
    Elderly subjects
    Highly sensitive patients
    Persons with dermographism
    Patients with widespread dermatoses
    Persons who do not like skin tests

Compared with skin-testing, RAST has some disadvantages that still do not permit its use on a large scale in clinical practice:

    High cost
    Results are delayed
    Requires purified allergens
    Requires trained technician, special laboratory equipment, and handling radioisotopes
    Does not detect non-IgE-mediated allergy (a new IgG RAST is developed)

Specific antibodies of other immunoglobulin classes can be measured by means of techniques similar to RAST. Toivanen and co-workers[73] measured IgM and IgG antibodies to cow's milk by radioimmunoassay with greater specificity and reproducibility than with the hemagglutination method. They concluded, however, that because of the high sensitivity of radioimmunoassays and the frequency of IgG and IgM antibodies in healthy subjects, normal and abnormal states are often difficult to differentiate. IgD antibodies to milk proteins can also be detected, although the presence of high titers has not yet been related to milk allergy.[68,74]

Clearly, antibodies to cow's milk proteins of many, perhaps all, immunoglobulin classes and subclasses are detectable in the sera of healthy subjects when sensitive techniques are used. The task confronting both the investigator and the clinician is to identify and put into use tests that can discriminate between health and disease, and between normal and abnormal immunologic responses.

Enzyme-linked Immunosorbent Assay (ELISA)

ELISA is a method for measuring specific antibodies of different immunoglobulin classes by means of enzyme-labeled rather than radio-labeled antiimmunoglobulin. The technique was originally described by Engvall and Perlmann,[75] and has been applied by Hanson et al.[76] and Fällstrom et al.[77] in measuring IgE, IgG, IgM, and IgA antibodies to cow's milk protein. It does not require the use of radioisotopes and has a great deal of potential, particularly for use in laboratories where the expensive equipment needed for radioimmunoassays is not available. It also has the distinct advantage of a long shelf-life of the enzyme-linked reagent, which can be used for several years, whereas the half-life of the usual nucleotide, ^{125}I, is 2 months. As currently used, however, ELISA is about one-tenth as sensitive as corresponding radioimmunoassays and will require considerably more refining for tests to be developed that clearly separate the normal from the milk-sensitive person.

Fluorescent Immunosorbent Test

Bürgin-Wolff et al.[77a] described a fluorescent immunosorbent test for IgG, IgA or IgM antibodies to cow's milk proteins. The patient's serum is incubated with antigen-coated polyacrylamide agarose beads, then washed and rabbit antihuman IgG, IgA, or IgM is added. After incubation and washing, the adding of fluorescein-labeled goat anti-rabbit immunoglobulin will demonstrate the presence of antibodies of the corresponding immunoglobulin class. This test is of limited practical use; its result is difficult to quantitate, and is frequently positive in patients with gastrointestinal diseases other than milk allergy.[77]

Precipitation Test

Testing for precipitating antibodies is conveniently carried out by the double-diffusion in agar technique of Ouchterlony.[78] The antigen (skimmed milk or purified milk protein fractions) is usually put in the central well and patient's sera to be tested for antibody are put in peripheral wells. As antigen and antibody diffuse through the agar and react with one another, complexes form that appear as precipitate lines, one for each antigen and its corresponding precipitating antibody. These lines can be analyzed visually (Fig. 6-2). Though the technique is relatively simple and inexpensive, it requires considerable experience for proper interpretation. It is not available in most community laboratories. All conditions, such as the percent and amount of agarose used, distances between reservoirs, time of incubation, the use of positive and negative controls, and other variables, must be carefully standardized if comparable results are to be expected. Antibodies of the IgG or IgA class can be detected when present in concentrations of approximately 50 μg/ml or more and of IgM antibodies in concentrations of about 200 μg/ml.

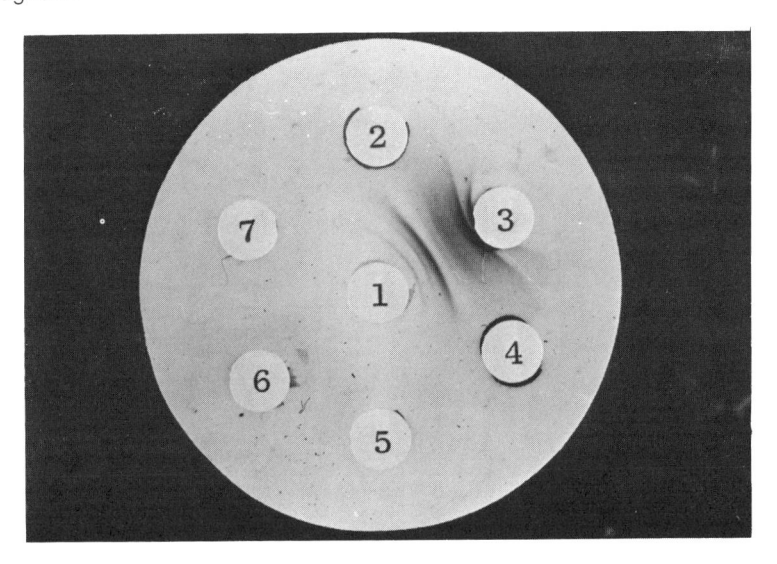

Fig. 6-2. Multiple precipitin lines between raw skim cow's milk diluted 1:10 (central reservoir) and serum from a patient with milk-induced chronic pulmonary disease (reservoir 3). Sera from two patients with other symptoms of milk allergy were placed in reservoirs 2 and 4. Reservoirs 5 and 6 contained sera from healthy nonallergic subjects, and reservoir 7 contained normal saline.

The sensitivity of the test is increased 10- to 20-fold by the use of Plexiglas reservoirs that allow the use of large amounts of reactants in relation to a thin layer of agar[79,80] (Fig. 6-3). Problems arise, however, because of binding of proteins to the reservoir wells, which, unless thoroughly cleaned or discarded after each test, may lead to false-negative results.

In one study of children with milk-induced gastrointestinal bleeding, antimilk precipitins were detected in 62 percent of patients, compared with 1 to 2 percent

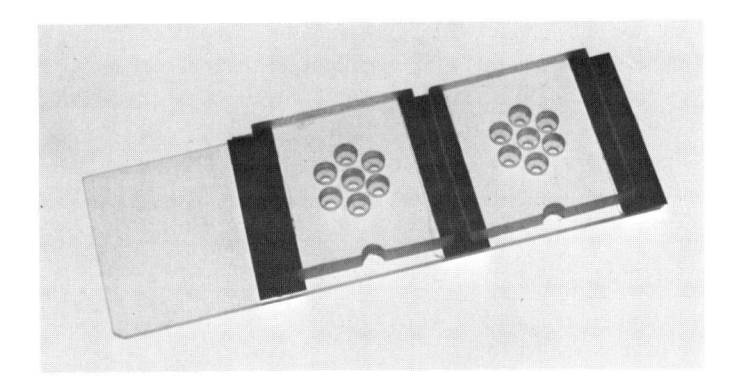

Fig. 6-3. Microslide technique of double diffusion in agar using Plexiglas reservoirs.

in an unselected population.[80] High precipitin titers or multiple precipitin bands are rare in normal persons[81,82] and are infrequent in adults with milk allergy.[83,84] In a group of children with chronic pulmonary disease of undetermined cause, a signficant number will have precipitins to cow's milk proteins in their sera.[11,74] If those with precipitins are then placed on a milk-free diet, a high percentage will vastly improve. This particular use of precipitin-in-agar tests has proved very useful over the years. The general use of precipitin tests to screen populations of allergic children, or even subjects suspected of milk-induced symptoms other than pulmonary disease or malabsorption, has not been rewarding.

A patient on a milk-free diet has a decrease in the precipitin titer usually within 2 to 4 months, and the titer may return to former levels after milk challenge.[47,85]

The titer of antimilk precipitins is increased in sera of patients with celiac disease, other chronic diarrheas, iron deficiency anemia, cystic fibrosis,[80] IgA deficiency, [86-88] Down's syndrome, [43,87,89] familial dysautonomia,[90,91] Wiskott-Aldrich syndrome, Hurler's syndrome, and chronic recurrent pneumonia.[92] The significance of antimilk precipitins in most of these conditions remains to be elucidated.

When a large series of sera containing antimilk precipitins was analyzed and compared with reference precipitate lines for ten specific cow's milk proteins, precipitins were usually directed to the heat-labile protein fractions that are present in small amounts.[93] That finding was somewhat unexpected, because heat-stable protein fractions, particularly beta-lactoglobulin and casein, were present in much greater quantity and appeared to be more allergenic than the heat-labile fractions in patients with milk-related intestinal malabsorption and diarrhea.

Coproantibodies.

Testing for fecal antibodies or coproantibodies to cow's milk has been carried out by the double-diffusion technique. The fecal extract is centrifuged and the supernatant is used. The stools should be fresh and processed as rapidly as possible. Results are less reproducible and less reliable than results of testing serum. False-positive results are frequent because of the formation of nonspecific deposits that resemble antigen-antibody precipitates. Also, the digestion of antibodies in the gut or in the specimen before it is tested will lead to false-negative results.

Although coproantibodies to milk have been noted in children with gastrointestinal milk allergy, sometimes without detectable antibodies in the serum,[94,95] they are probably not reliable indicators of milk allergy because they are also frequently present in patients with nonspecific diarrheas.[96]

Hemagglutination Test

Passive hemagglutination techniques using antigen-coated erythrocytes (rabbit, sheep, or group 0 human erythrocytes) are sensitive tests for detecting specific antibodies of the IgM or IgG classes. IgM antibody is about 750 times as efficient as IgG in agglutination.[97] The antigen (skimmed cow's milk or isolated protein fractions) is coupled to the surface of erythrocytes by the tannic acid[98] or the bisdiazodized benzidine technique.[99]

Antimilk hemagglutinins seem to be of even less help than precipitins in verifying the diagnosis of milk allergy, because they are so common in normal persons.[92,98,100,101] High titers, however, suggest an abnormal response, and have been noted in about one-half to three-fourths of sera from patients with milk allergy.[31,41,42,58,102] High titers are more frequent in infants and children than in older people.[103] The titer decreases after milk elimination, and increases on challenge.[102,103]

High titers of antimilk hemagglutinins have been reported in some patients with ulcerative colitis,[104,105] Down's syndrome,[89] sudden infant-death syndrome,[106] Wiskott-Aldrich syndrome,[107] familial dysautonomia,[91] myocardial infarction,[108] and in a variety of chronic diseases.[92] Their role in the pathogenesis of these diseases has never been clarified.

Complement-fixation Test

The fixation of complement by antigen-antibody complexes can also be used as a sensitive measure of specific IgG and IgM antibodies. The basis of this test is the measurement of reduced complement activity in the presence of antigen-antibody complexes. Antigen and antibody are incubated with a known amount of complement; then the remaining complement activity is measured by adding a suspension of sensitized sheep erythrocytes and observing for hemolysis. The degree of lysis depends on the amount of free active complement and is inversely proportional to the amount of immune complexes present. The use of this test in the detection of antibodies to cow's milk protein has not achieved popularity. In some instances, the test reaction was positive in the absence of detectable antimilk precipitins,[109] a result that is not surprising because of the greater sensitivity of the complement-fixation reaction. Its usefulness is probably similar to the hemagglutination test in the detection of antibodies to milk proteins,[110] although it is perhaps slightly less sensitive than that test.

Immune Complexes

The presence of circulating immune complexes involving milk antigens has been reported in a high percentage of infants after the ingestion of cow's milk.[111] Indeed, immune complexes are probably normally present in small amounts in all people. Different tests for circulating complexes have differing degrees of sensitivity and may measure different kinds of complexes.[97,112,113] No single technique is completely reliable. Raji cell radioimmunoassay and Clq binding assays seem to be among the best. What is now needed is the development of tests that will measure normal circulating immune complexes separately from those that have pathogenetic significance. Thus, although tests for circulating complexes involving milk antigens may eventually prove helpful, they are presently of little value to the clinician.

Leukocyte Histamine Release

The leukocyte histamine release test is a useful indicator of immediate-type hypersensitivity to foods.[114,115] Peripheral leukocytes (basophils) are mixed in vitro with the allergen under consideration, and the amount of histamine released is expressed as a percentage of the total histamine in the leukocytes. The percentage must be compared with that of histamine released spontaneously from cells not exposed to the antigen. Leukocytes of children allergic to foods may even show an increased in vitro release of histamine without the addition of any antigen.[16] The test is not completely specific and is not practical for routinely diagnosing milk allergy.[28,116]

Cytotoxic Food Test

When the leukocytes of a food-sensitive patient are incubated with the offending antigen, the cells may become nonmotile and round, and then lyse. This test was origianlly described by Black in 1956[117] and later modified by Bryan and Bryan.[118] The test is presently impractical for diagnosing food allergy. It has too many false-positive and false-negative results, it is not a quantitative procedure, and subjective interpretations are required. At present, its correlation with clinical disease is rather poor. Nevertheless, the test may show promise when these difficulties have been overcome because cells from allergic subjects are more likely to show changes in leukocyte morphology when exposed to an antigen than are cells of nonallergic subjects. Measurements of antigen-induced changes in cell metabolism or function, or of specifically released chemicals would appear worthy of investigation.

Lymphoblast Transformation Test

The in vitro antigen-induced lymphocyte stimulation procedure has been used in recent years in studies of patients with milk allergy. Cultures of the patient's peripheral blood lymphocytes are prepared, and predetermined amounts of skim milk or isolated milk proteins are added. Control cultures must be tested, including unstimulated lymphocytes, lymphocytes stimulated by mitogens, and antigen stimulation of lymphocytes of healthy subjects. Tritiated thymidine is added on the fifth day, and a day later the lymphocytes are harvested. The counts of incorporated radioactivity indicate the amount of DNA that is synthesized, which is taken as a measure of lymphocyte proliferation. The degree of antigen-induced proliferation is indicated by the ratio of the count of the antigen-stimulated culture to the mean count of unstimulated cultures. The incorporated counts from mitogen-stimulated cultures indicate maximal degrees of incorporation; they demonstrate as well the viability of the cells.

A high reliability for the test has been reported by some,[119-121] but not by others.[116] Lymphocytes of allergic patients may show an increased proliferation in vitro without the addition of the specific antigen.[122] Another limitation of the test is that beta-lactoglobulin preparations may have a significant nonspecific mitogenic activity even on lymphocytes of normal subjects.[123]

Lymphokine Production

Ashkenazi and co-workers[123a] found that when lymphocytes from milk-sensitive patients were stimulated in vitro by cow's milk protein, their production of leukocyte migration inhibition factor was several fold higher than in controls, and with the disappearance of milk-sensitivity the production of leukocyte migration inhibition declines.

INTESTINAL BIOPSY

The histopathology of the gastrointestinal tract in milk allergy was discussed in some detail earlier (Chap. 5). Based on the observation that oral milk challenge may induce mucosal changes in the absence of clinical symptoms,[57, 124, 125] some workers[57] have advocated the use of small-bowel biopsy as the critical diagnostic procedure in milk allergy. Nevertheless, since many forms of extraintestinal milk allergy and even milk-induced diarrhea can occur in the absence of abnormal jejunal histopathology, and since the histologic changes in the intestinal mucosa are nonspecific[126] and inconsistent,[50] the routine histologic examination by light microscopy in all suspected cases of milk allergy cannot be recommended. On the other hand, valuable research information may be obtained from immunofluorescence studies of the intestinal mucosal biopsy specimen. Ideally, a peroral jejunal biopsy specimen is obtained before oral milk challenge, and sequentially at intervals afterward. The mucosa may show an increase in the number of immunoglobulin- or complement-bearing immunocytes,[57, 124, 127] as well as other changes (see Chap. 5). Duodenal mucosal biopsy specimens from milk-sensitive patients have also shown increased numbers of eosinophils infiltrating the lamina propria.[128]

REFERENCES

1. Clein NW: Cow's milk allergy in infants. Pediatr Clin North Am 4:949–962, 1954
2. Buisseret PD: Common manifestations of cow's milk allergy in children. Lancet 1:304–305, 1978
3. Randolph TG: Dynamics, diagnosis, and treatment of food allergy. Otolaryngol Clin North Am 7:617–635, 1974
4. Gerrard JW: Familial recurrent rhinorrhea and bronchitis due to cow's milk. JAMA 198:605–607, 1966
5. Gerrard JW, Heiner DC, Ives EJ, et al.: Milk allergy: Recognition, natural history and management. Clin Pediatr 2:634–641, 1963
6. Gerrard JW, Lubos MC, Hardy LW, et al.: Milk allergy: Clinical picture and familial incidence. Can Med Assoc J 97:780–785, 1967
7. Speer F: Food allergy: The 10 common offenders. Am Fam Physician 13:106–112, 1976
8. Deamer WC: Recurrent abdominal pain: A frequent manifestation of food allergy. Curr Med Dialog 40:130–154, 1973
9. Gerrard JW: Allergy in infancy. Pediatr Ann 3:9–23, 1974
10. Coe B, Mansmann HC Jr: Similar multiple milk protein intolerances in non-fraternal twins. Ann Allergy 24:307–308, 1966
11. Heiner DC, Sears JW, Kniker WT: Multiple precipitins to cow's milk in chronic respiratory disease. Am J Dis Child 103:634–654, 1962
12. Vendel S: Cow's milk idiosyncrasy in infants. Acta Paediatr Scand (Suppl 5) 35:3–37, 1948
13. Goldman AS, Anderson DW, Jr, Sellers WA, et al.: Milk Allergy. I. Oral challenge with milk and isolated milk proteins in allergic children. Pediatrics 32:425–443, 1963
14. Gryboski JD: Gastrointestinal milk allergy in infants. Pediatrics 40:354–362, 1967
15. Walker-Smith JA: Gastrointestinal allergy. Practitioner 220:562–573, 1978
16. May CD: Objective clinical and laboratory studies of immediate hypersensitivity reactions to foods in asthmatic children. J Allergy Clin Immunol 58:500–515, 1976
17. Bock SA, Lee WY, Remigio LK, et al.: Studies of hypersensitivity reactions to foods in infants and children. J Allergy Clin Immunol 62:327–334, 1978
18. Loveless MH: Milk allergy: A survey of its incidence; experiments with a masked ingestion test. J Allergy 21:489–499, 1950
19. Pfeiffer GO: Sublingual procedures. Trans Am Soc Ophthalmol Otolaryngol Allergy 11:104–107, 1970
20. Dickey LD: Ecologic illness: Investigations by provocative tests with foods and chemicals, 1963-1970. Rocky Mt Med J 68:23–28, 1971
21. Breneman JC, Hurst A, Heiner DC, et al.: Final report of the food allergy committee of the American College of Allergists on the clinical evaluation of sublingual provocative testing method for diagnosis of food allergy. Ann Allergy 33:164–166, 1974
22. Rinkle HJ, Lee CH, Brown DW, et al.: The diagnosis of food allergy. Arch Otolaryngol 79:71–79, 1964
23. Caplin I: Report of the committee on provocative food testing. Ann Allergy 31:375–381, 1973
24. Crawford LV, Lieberman P, Harfi HA, et al.: A double-blind study of subcutaneous food testing sponsored by the Food Committee of the American Academy of Allergy. J Allergy Clin Immunol 57:236, 1976
25. Bachman KD, Dees SC: Milk allergy. II. Observations on incidence and symptoms of allergy to milk in allergic infants. Pediatrics 20:400–407, 1957
26. Saperstein S, Anderson DW: Antigenicity of milk proteins of prepared formulas measured by precipitin ring test and passive cutaneous anaphylaxis in the guinea pig. J Pediatr 61:196–204, 1962

27. Mueller HL, Weiss RJ, O'Leary D, et al.: The incidence of milk sensitivity and the development of allergy in infants. N Engl J Med 268:1220–1224, 1963
28. Galant SP, Bullock J, Frick OL: An immunological approach to the diagnosis of food sensitivity. Clin Allergy 3:363–372, 1973
29. Bullock JD, Bodenbender JG: A simple laboratory aid in diagnosing food allergy. Ann Allergy 28:127–132, 1970
30. Gavani UD, Hyde JS, Moore BS: Hypersensitivity to milk and egg white: Skin tests, RAST results and clinical intolerance. Ann Allergy 40:314–318, 1978
31. Oehling A, Martin-Gil D, Jeréz J, et al.: "In vitro" diagnosis of food allergy. Allergol Immunopathol (Madr) 6:153–161, 1978
32. Norman PS, Marsh DG: Human serum albumin and Tween 80 as stabilizers of allergen solutions. J Allergy Clin Immunol 62:314–319, 1978
33. Bleumink E, Berrens L: Synthetic approaches to the biological activity of β-lactoglobulin in human allergy to cow's milk. Nature (London) 212:541–543, 1966
34. Lietze A: Laboratory research in food allergy. I. Food allergens. J Asthma Res 7:25–40, 1969
35. Spies JR, Stevan MA, Stein WJ, et al.: The chemistry of allergens. XX. New antigens generated by pepsin hydrolysis of bovine milk proteins. J Allergy 45:208–219, 1970
36. Matthews TS, Soothill JF: Complement activation after milk feeding in children with cow's milk allergy. Lancet 2:893–895, 1970
37. Rebuck JW, Crowley JH: A method of studying leukocyte function in vivo. Ann NY Acad Sci 59:757–794, 1955
38. Ishizaka K, Ishizaka T, Hornbrook MM: Physico-chemical properties of reaginic antibody. IV. Presence of a unique immunoglobulin as a carrier of reaginic activity. J Immunol 97:75–85, 1966
39. Wide L, Bennich H, Johansson SGO: Diagnosis of allergy by an in-vitro test for allergen antibodies. Lancet 2:1105–1107, 1967
40. Bazaral M, Orgel HA, Hamburger RN: The influence of serum IgE levels of selected recipients, including patients with allergy, helminthiasis and tuberculosis, on the apparent P-K titer of a reaginic serum. Clin Exp Immunol 14:117–125, 1973
41. Baudon JJ, Fontaine JL, Mougenot JF, et al.: Digestive intolerance to cow's milk proteins in infants. Biological and histological study. Arch Fr Pediatr 32:787–801, 1975
42. Fontaine JL, Navarro J: Small intestinal biopsy in cow's milk protein allergy in infancy. Arch Dis Child 50:357–362, 1975
43. Kuitunen P, Visakorpi JK, Savilahti E, et al.: Malabsorption syndrome with cow's milk intolerance. Arch Dis Child 50:351–356, 1975
44. Ottesen EA, Cohen SG: The eosinophil, eosinophilia and eosinophil-related disorders, in Middleton E, Jr, Reed CE, Ellis EF (eds): Allergy Principles and Practice, vol II. St. Louis, Mosby, 1978, pp 584–632
45. Beeson PB, Bass DA: The Eosinophil. Philadelphia, Saunders, 1977, pp 161–189
46. Waldmann TA, Wochner RD, Laster L, et al.: Allergic gastroenteropathy: A cause of excessive gastrointestinal protein loss. N Engl J Med 276:761–769, 1967
47. Silver H, Douglas DM: Milk intolerance in infancy. Arch Dis Child 43:17–22, 1968
48. Osvath P, Markus M: Diagnostic value of thrombopenia and eosinophilia after food ingestion in children with milk and egg allergy. Acta Paediatr Acad Sci Hung 9:279–284, 1968
49. Lebenthal E, Laor J, Lewitus Z, et al.: Gastrointestinal protein loss in allergy to cow's milk β-lactoglobulin. Isr J Med Sci 6:506–510, 1970
50. Iyngkaran N, Robinson MJ, Prathap K, et al.: Cow's milk protein-sensitive enteropathy: Combined clinical and histological criteria for diagnosis. Arch Dis Child 53:20–26, 1978
51. Nance FD: Stool eosinophilia in gastrointestinal allergy of infants. J Pediatr 33:313–317, 1948
52. Hansel FK: Clinical Allergy. St. Louis, Mosby, 1953, p 411

53. Fineman SM, Rosen FS, Geha RS: Transient hypogammaglobulinemia, elevated immunoglobulin E level, and food allergy. J Allergy Clin Immunol 64:216–222, 1979
54. Gleich GJ, Averbeck AK, Swedlund HA: Measurement of IgE in normal and allergic serum by radioimmunoassay. J Lab Clin Med 77:690–698, 1971
55. Ceska M, Lundkvist V: A new and simple radioimmunoassay method for the determination of IgE. Immunochemistry 9:1021–1030, 1972
56. Boat TF, Polmar SH, Whitman V, et al.: Hyperreactivity to cow milk in young children with pulmonary hemosiderosis and cor pulmonale secondary to nasopharyngeal obstruction. J Pediatr 87:23–29, 1975
57. Shiner M, Ballard J, Brook CGD, et al.: Intestinal biopsy in the diagnosis of cow's milk protein intolerance without acute symptoms. Lancet 2:1060–1063, 1975
58. Subira ML, Oehling A, Crisci CD, et al.: Evaluation of total IgE in diverse allergosis. Comparative study with other techniques. Part II. Allergol Immunopathol (Madr) 4:51–66, 1976
59. Heiner DC, Rose B: Elevated levels of IgE (γE) in conditions other than classical atopy. J Allergy 45:30–42, 1970
60. Johansson SGO, Bennich H, Berg T: The clinical significance of IgE. Prog Clin Immunol 1:157–181, 1972
61. Nordbring F, Johansson SGO, Espmark A: Raised serum levels of IgE in infectious mononucleosis. Scand J Infect Dis 4:119–124, 1972
62. Kusakawa S, Heiner DC: Elevated levels of immunoglobulin E in the acute febrile mucocutaneous lymph node syndrome. Pediatr Res 10:108–111, 1976
63. Bahna SL, Horwitz CA, Heiner DC: IgE in cytomegalovirus mononucleosis. J Allergy Clin Immunol 61:177, 1978
64. Bahna SL, Horwitz CA, Fiala M, Heiner DC: IgE response in heterophil-positive infectious mononucleosis. J Allergy Clin Immunol 62:167–173, 1978
65. Hoffman DR, Haddad ZH: Diagnosis of IgE mediated reactions to food antigens by radioimmunoassay. J Allergy Clin Immunol 54:165–173, 1974
66. Aas K: The diagnosis of hypersensitivity to ingested foods. Clin Allergy 8:39–50, 1978
67. Haddad ZH, Kalra V, Verma S: IgE antibodies to peptic and peptic-tryptic digests of beta-lactoglobulin: Significance in food hypersensitivity. Ann Allergy 42:368–371, 1979
68. Bahna SL, Tateno K, Heiner DC: Elevated IgD antibodies to wheat in celiac disease. Ann Allergy 44:—, 1980
69. Foucard T: A follow-up study of children with asthmatoid bronchitis. Acta Paediatr Scand 62:633–644, 1973
70. Wütrich B, Kopper E: Determination of specific IgE serum antibodies using the radioallergosorbent-test (RAST) and its significance for the diagnosis of atopic allergy. Schweiz Med Wochenschr 105:1337–1345, 1975
71. Lowenstein H, Krasilnikoff PA, Bjerrum OJ, et al.: Occurrence of specific precipitins against bovine whey proteins in serum from children with gastrointestinal disorders. Int Arch Allergy Appl Immunol 55:514–525, 1977
72. Turner KJ, Sumarmo, Matondang-Siahaan C: Precipitating factors in respiratory allergic disease in Indonesian children. Clin Allergy 8:145–154, 1978
73. Toivanen A, Viljanen MK, Savilahti E: IgM and IgG anti-milk antibodies measured by radioimmunoassay in myocardial infarction. Lancet 2:205–207, 1975
74. Lee SK, Kniker WT, Cook CD, Heiner DC: Cow's milk induced pulmonary disease in children, in Barness LA (ed): Advances in Pediatrics, vol 25. Chicago, Year Book, 1978, pp 39–57
75. Engvall E, Perlmann P: Enzyme-linked immunosorbent assay, ELISA. III. Quantitation of specific antibodies by enzyme-labelled anti-immunoglobulin in antigen coated tubes. J Immunol 109:129–135, 1972
76. Hanson LÅ, Ahlstedt S, Carlsson B, et al.: Secretory IgA antibodies against cow's milk

proteins in human milk and their possible effect in mixed feeding. Int Arch Allergy Appl Immunol 54:457–462, 1977
77. Fällström SP, Ahlstedt S, Hanson LÅ: Specific antibodies in infants with gastrointestinal intolerance to cow's milk protein. Int Arch Allergy Appl Immunol 56:97–105, 1978
77a. Bürgin-Wolff A, Hernandez R, Just M: A rapid fluorescent solid-phase method for detecting antibodies against milk proteins and gliadin in different immunoglobulin classes. Experientia (Basel) 28:119–120, 1972
77b. Signer E, Bürgin–Wolff A, Berger R, et al.: Antibodies to gliadin as a screening test for coeliac disease: A prospective study. Helv Paediatr Acta 34:41–52, 1979
78. Ouchterlony O: Antigen-antibody reactions in gel. IV. Types of reactions in coordinated systems of diffusion. Acta Pathol Microbiol Scand 32:231– 240, 1953
79. Crowle AJ: A simplified micro double-diffusion agar precipitation technique. J Lab Clin Med 52:784–787, 1958
80. Heiner DC, Lahey ME, Wilson JF, et al.: Precipitins to antigens of wheat and cow's milk in celiac disease. J Pediatr 61:813–830, 1962
81. Heiner DC, Sears JW: Chronic respiratory disease associated with multiple circulating precipitins to cow's milk. Am J Dis Child 100:500–502, 1960
82. Hinkle NH, Hong R, West CD: Identification of the antigen and symptomatology of children with precipitins to milk. Am J Dis Child 102:449–452, 1961
83. Bayless TM, Partin JS, Rosensweig NS: Absence of milk antibodies in milk intolerance in adults. JAMA 201:50, 1967
84. Jussila J: Milk intolerance and lactose malabsorption in hospital patients and young servicemen in Finland. Ann Clin Res 1:199–207, 1969
85. Heiner DC, Wilson JF, Lahey ME: Sensitivity to cow's milk. JAMA 189:563–567, 1964
86. Buckley RH, Dees SC: Correlation of milk precipitins with IgA deficiency. N Engl J Med 281:465–469, 1969
87. Huntley CC, Robbins JB, Lyerly AD, et al.: Characterization of precipitating antibodies to ruminant serum and milk proteins in humans with selective IgA deficiency. N Engl J Med 284:7–10, 1971
88. Barrett DJ, Bertani L, Wara DW, et al.: Milk precipitins in selective IgA deficiency. Ann Allergy 42:73–76, 1979
89. Nelson TL: Spontaneously occurring milk antibodies in mongoloids. Am J Dis Child 108: 494–498, 1964
90. Drucker M, Russel A, Kletter B, et al.: Milk antibodies in familial dysautonomia. Pediatrics 44:265–268, 1969
91. Shapira E, Tenebaum R, Kletter B, et al: Definition of cow's milk protein fraction evoking precipitating antibodies. J Lab Clin Med 77:529– 534, 1971
92. Peterson RDA, Good RA: Antibodies to cow's milk proteins: Their presence and significance. Pediatrics 31:209–221, 1963
93. Bahna SL, Heiner DC: Cow's milk allergy: Pathogenesis, manifestations, diagnosis and management, in Barness LA (ed): Advances in Pediatrics, vol 25. Chicago, Year Book, 1978, pp 1–37
94. Katz J, Spiro HM, Herskovic T: Milk precipitating substance in the stool in gastrointestinal milk sensitivity. N Engl J Med 278:1191–1194, 1968
95. Gryboski JD, Katz J, Reynolds D, et al.: Gluten intolerance following cow's milk sensitivity: Two cases with coproantibodies to milk and wheat proteins. Ann Allergy 26:33–39, 1968
96. Davis SD, Bierman CW, Pierson WE, et al.: Clinical nonspecificity of milk coproantibodies in diarrheal stools. N Engl J Med 282:612–613, 1970
97. Stites DP: Clinical laboratory methods for detection of antigens and antibodies, in Fudenberg HH, Stites DP, Caldwell JI, et al. (eds): Basic and Clinical Immunology. Los Altos, Calif., Lange, Publications, 1978, p 337–374

98. Gunther M, Aschaffenburg R, Matthews RH, et al.: The level of antibodies to the proteins of cow's milk in the serum of normal human infants. Immunology 3:296–306, 1960
99. Gordon J, Rose B, Sehon AH: Detection of "non-precipitating" antibodies in sera of individuals allergic to ragweed pollen by an in vitro method. J Exp Med 108:37–51, 1958
100. Collins-Williams C, Salama Y: A laboratory study on the diagnosis of milk allergy. Int Arch Allergy 27:110–128, 1965
101. Dees SC: Some unresolved problems in clinical allergy: Observations on milk and egg hemagglutinating antibody titers in allergic children. Pediatrics 50:420–428, 1972
102. Sobien-Kopczynska S, Denys A, Mazur-Cybulska J: Passive hemagglutination test in detection of hypersensitivity to cow's milk in children with recurrent spastic bronchitis and pneumonia. Bull Pol Med Sci Hist 13:120–123, 1970
103. Matsumura T, Kuroume T, Tajima S: Acetonemic vomiting from viewpoint of food allergy. Acta Allergol 25:423–450, 1970
104. Davidson L: Milk proteins in ulcerative colitis. Br Med J 2:1358, 1961
105. Taylor KB, Truelove SC: Circulating antibodies to milk proteins in ulcerative colitis. Br Med J 2:924–929, 1961
106. Parish WE, Richards CB, France NE, et al.: Further investigations on the hypothesis that some cases of cot-death are due to a modified anaphylactic reaction to cow's milk. Int Arch Allergy 24:215–243, 1964
107. Hunter A, Feinstein A, Coombs RRA: Immunoglobulin class of antibodies to cow's milk casein in infant sera and evidence for low molecular weight IgM antibodies. Immunology 15:381–388, 1968
108. Davies DF, Johnson AP, Rees BWG, et al.: Food antibodies and myocardial infarction. Lancet 1:1012–1014, 1974
109. Parish WE: Detection of reaginic and short-term sensitizing anaphylactic or anaphylactoid antibodies to milk in sera of allergic and normal persons. Clin Allergy 1:369–380, 1971
110. Oehling A, Subira ML: The Boyden and complement fixation test in diagnosis of allergic diseases. Allergol Immunopathol (Madr) 1:3–10, 1973
111. Delire M, Cambiaso CL, Masson PL: Circulating immune complexes in infants fed on cow's milk. Nature (London) 272:632, 1978
112. Kohler PF: Immune complexes and allergic disease, in Middleton E, Jr, Reed CE, Ellis EF (eds): Allergy Principles and Practice, Vol I. St. Louis, Mosby, 1978, pp 155–176
113. Gubler RH, Lambert PH: Detection of immune complexes in human diseases. Prog Allergy 24:1–48, 1978
114. Golbert TM, Patterson R, Pruzansky JJ: Systemic allergic reactions to ingested antigens. J Allergy 44:96–107, 1969
115. May CE, Lyman M, Alberto R, et al.: Procedures for immunochemical study of histamine release from leukocytes with small volume of blood. J Allergy 46:12–20, 1970
116. May CE, Alberto R: In-vitro responses of leucocytes to food proteins in allergic and normal children: Lymphocyte stimulation and histamine release. Clin Allergy 2:335–344, 1972
117. Black AP: A new diagnostic method in allergic disease. Pediatrics 17:716–724, 1956
118. Bryan WTK, Bryan MP: Cytology in otolaryngology. Trans Am Acad Ophthalmol Otolaryngol 63:597–612, 1959
119. Endré L, Osvath P: Antigen-induced lymphoblast transformation in the diagnosis of cow's milk allergic diseases in infancy and early childhood. Acta Allergol (Kbh) 30:34–42, 1975
120. Scheinmann P, Gendrel D, Charles J, et al.: Value of lymphoblast transformation test in cow's milk protein intestinal intolerance. Clin Allergy 6:515–521, 1976
121. Stafford HA, Polmar SH, Boat TF: Immunologic studies in cow's milk-induced pulmonary hemosiderosis. Pediatr Res 11:898–903, 1977
122. May CD, Alberto R: In vivo stimulation of peripheral lymphocytes to proliferation after oral challenge of children allergic to foods. Int Arch Allergy Appl Immunol 43:525–532, 1972

123. Asquith P, Housley J, Cooke WT: Lymphocyte stimulation by bovine β-lactoglobulin. Nature (London) 228:462–464, 1970
123a. Ashkenazi A, Levin S, Ider D, et al.: An immunological assay for sensitivity to cow's milk protein. X International Congress of Allergology, Jerusalem, Nov., 4–11, 1979
124. Savilahti E: Immunochemical study of the malabsorption syndrome with cow's milk intolerance. Gut 14:491–501, 1973
125. Vitoria JC, Aranjuelo ME, Rodriguez-Soriano J: Jejunal biopsy in cow's milk protein intolerance. Lancet 1:722–723, 1978
126. Kilby A, Walker-Smith JA, Wood CBS: Small intestinal mucosa in cow's milk allergy. Lancet 1:531, 1975
127. Harris MJ, Petts V, Penny R: Cow's milk allergy as a cause of infantile colic: Immunofluorescent studies on jejunal mucosa. Aust Paediatr J 13:276–281, 1977
128. Withrington R, Challacombe DN: Eosinophil-counts in duodenal tissue in cow's milk allergy. Lancet 1:675, 1979

7
Differential Diagnosis

No single manifestation of cow's milk allergy is by itself pathognomonic of the condition. Symptoms identical to those of milk allergy may be caused by a wide variety of acute or chronic disorders. Overzealous diagnosis of milk allergy might result in overlooking a more serious disease. Because providing a comprehensive differential diagnosis of all manifestations of milk allergy would be impractical, the following discussion will be limited to the more important conditions that should be considered when the possibility of milk allergy involving the gastrointestinal tract, the respiratory tract, or the skin exists.

Besides thorough history-taking and a careful physical examination, selected laboratory diagnostic studies may help considerably. The elimination of cow's milk, however, need not be delayed until all investigations have been completed. In fact, improvement on a milk-free diet may obviate unnecessary procedures.

OTHER ALLERGENS

As should be kept in mind, the patient's symptoms may be caused by allergens other than, or in addition to, milk. Because few, if any, symptoms are unique to milk allergy, allergies to other ingestants, inhalants, or contactants must always be considered. Egg, chocolate, cereal, grains, corn, orange, tomato, meat, fish, nuts, vitamin preparations, drugs, and food additives are rather frequent ingestant allergens, in both children and adults. They belong to the list of suspect allergens, the intake of which should be carefully regulated during "elimination-challenge tests." All foods taken during these procedures should be

ALLERGY TO FOREIGN SUBSTANCES IN COW'S MILK

In some instances, allergic symptoms follow the ingestion of cow's milk but are caused by pollutants rather than by normal milk constituents. Extrinsic allergens that may be present in raw cow's milk, either by adulteration or by accidental pollution, probably include wheat, peanut, linseed, cottonseed, ragweed, primula, and bacteria,[1] and antibiotics, hormones, and other drugs occasionally administered to cattle. Symptoms such as headache, fatigue, tremor, and collapse have been attributed to the ingestion of milk from cows that have eaten a certain type of weed called white snakeroot *(Eupatorium rugosum)*.[2]

Penicillin, a potent drug allergen, is frequently used to treat bovine mastitis, and milk distributors have occasionally added it to milk as a preservative. Because milk containing penicillin constitutes a health hazard to penicillin-sensitive persons, the United States Food and Drug Administration in 1953 prohibited the sale of milk from cows being treated with penicillin. It also prohibited the adding of pencillin to milk.[3] In spite of those rules, however, allergic reactions resulting from penicillin contained in milk continued to be reported.[4,5] Wicher and co-workers[6] documented, in a woman known to be highly sensitive to penicillin, a severe allergic reaction after ingestion of milk that was found to contain the drug in a concentration of approximately 10 U/ml.

GASTROINTESTINAL DISORDERS

Gastrointestinal symptoms during childhood may result from a wide variety of conditions. Malabsorption syndromes deserve special consideration because of the need for early recognition and appropriate management.[7,8] Conditions that may be confused with milk allergy include the following:

Improper Feeding Habits

Gastrointestinal upsets in infants are frequently caused by poor feeding practices such as overfeeding, too early introduction of solid foods, or feeding excessive quantities of new foods. Not uncommonly, an inexperienced or ill-informed mother will force her child to take a certain amount of formula at every feeding regardless of the child's appetite. The feeding of too concentrated a formula may result in loose, frequent stools. Too much fat delays gastric emptying and causes distention and abdominal discomfort. A diet too rich in carbohydrate may lead to fermentation in the bowel, distention, flatulence, and loose stools. The underfed infant may cry excessively, be irritable, fail to thrive, be apathetic, and have constipation or "starvation" diarrhea. Swallowing air during feeding from the bottle is a common cause of abdominal distention, discomfort, and excessive regurgitation. Vomiting, colic, and irritability in young infants are frequently related to maternal emotional instability or to a tense social environment.

To dispel maternal worry and stress on the infant, many mothers need reassurance that normal infants, especially during the first 6 months of life, commonly "spit up" or regurgitate small quantities of formula shortly after feeding.

Food Additives

Artificial colors and flavors are so widely used in foods and beverages, that they are ingested almost daily by most inhabitants of industrialized countries. Many adverse reactions to food additives have been reported.[9,10] The yellow dye tartrazine in particular has come under recent scrutiny, so much so that the United States Food and Drug Administration has recommended that all medication given to allergic subjects should be free of this coloring agent. Perhaps this recommendation should be extended to the use of all unnecessary chemical dyes and additives in medicines and foods. At least the quantites now used, which are largely unregulated, could be greatly reduced.

Lactose Intolerance

In lactose intolerance, stools may be frequent, watery, and acidic, and have an increased content of reducing sugar because of an inability to split the disaccharide lactose adequately. A lactase deficiency in the small intestinal mucosa is accompanied by an abnormal lactose tolerance test. Gastrointestinal milk allergy may be difficult to distinguish from lactase deficiency because both conditions improve when casein hydrolysate or lactose-free soy formulas are substituted for cow's milk.

Congenital lactase deficiency is rare, and is manifested in the newborn by frequent, watery, acidic stools, whether the baby is bottle-fed or breast-fed, because both types of milk contain lactose. Acquired lactase deficiency is more common, and occurs secondary to a variety of gastrointestinal disorders including gastroenteritis, celiac disease, gastrointestinal allergy, chronic nonspecific diarrhea, and the prolonged intake of certain medications.[11,12] Secondary deficiency is transient and may last for a few days to several weeks after recovery from the primaary condition or removal of the offending agent. A developmental form of lactase deficiency occurs in adults, and has an incidence of about 70 percent in adult blacks, Asians, and Jews.[11] Transient lactose intolerance occurs in more than 50 percent of patients with severe gastrointestinal milk allergy, and may persist for several weeks after milk elimination.[13-19] Some commercial preparations of lactose are derived from cow's milk and have been found to be contaminated with milk protein.[20]

Celiac Disease

Celiac disease or gluten-induced enteropathy may be difficult to differentiate from milk-induced gastroenteropathy. Both may cause malabsorption, steatorrhea, hypoproteinemia, microcytic hypochronic anemia, growth retardation, and changes in the intestinal mucosa.[21] Precipitins to milk proteins may be present in both diseases.[22,23] Celiac disease becomes manifest after a critical amount of wheat gluten has been introduced in the diet, the amount that will result in overt celiac disease varies from person to person. The amount of ingested cow's milk that will result in a milk-related celiac-like syndrome in susceptible subjects also varies from patient to patient. Diagnosis of either condition depends on finding a flat mucosa in the small bowel, and seeing a dramatic clinical and histologic improvement if gluten or milk is eliminated. Several studies showed that patients with milk allergy later developed celiac disease,[24-27] further attesting to a similarity in the pathogenesis of the two conditions.

Cystic Fibrosis

Either gastrointestinal or respiratory symptoms of cystic fibrosis, or both, may appear during infancy or early childhood, and often the disease is initially misdiagnosed as milk allergy. The symptoms, however, have little relation to the antigenic constituents of the diets. In addition to pancreatic dysfunction, a deficiency in intestinal lactase is common.[28] Cystic fibrosis should be suspected if a child who has a family history of cystic fibrosis has intestinal malfunction, growth retardation, or pulmonary symptoms, or in a child without a family history of the disease, if the child has characteristic frequent, large, foul-smelling stools, especially with concomitant pulmonary pathology. The diagnosis is established by demonstrating an increase in the concentrations of sodium and chloride in sweat, and, in cases in which these studies are equivocal, by demonstrating absent pancreatic enzymes and an increased viscosity in the duodenal juice.

Shwachman Syndrome

Shwachman and co-workers[29] described a syndrome consisting of pancreatic insufficiency and bone marrow hypoplasia. In addition to gastrointestinal symptoms, signs of the disease include neutropenia and occasionally anemia and thrombocytopenia. There is no pulmonary disease, and the sweat chloride test shows normal results.

Galactosemia

Galactosemia is an extremely rare disease that is caused by a deficiency in the galactose-1-phosphatase uridyl transferase or one of the galactokinase enzymes. The affected infant has severe gastrointestinal symptoms, galactosemia, galactosuria, and cataracts. If fed cow's milk, the child may die quickly. Feeding a protein hydrolysate or a galactose-free diet is essential. The diagnosis is verified by measuring the specific enzymes in the erythrocytes.

Sucrose Intolerance

The gastrointestinal symptoms of sucrose intolerance appear when sucrose in any form is introduced into the diet. It is a rare condition and is caused by the deficiency of the enzyme sucrase-isomaltase. The diagnosis is verified by a sucrose tolerance test.

Enterokinase Deficiency

Deficiency of the enterokinase enzyme is also a rare disease that may be misdiagnosed as cow's milk allergy because the patient may tolerate casein hydrolysate but not ordinary cow's milk formula. Amylase and lipase are quantitatively normal but their enzymatic activity is extremely low because of the lack of enterokinase. The deficiency can be detected by testing the duodenal aspirate.

Congenital Chloridorrhea

Defective absorption of chloride is a rare familial disease. Unabsorbed chloride may result in an increase in intraluminal osmotic pressure, watery diarrhea, and excessive loss of electrolytes. A high stool chloride in association with a low level of serum chloride confirms the diagnosis.

Ulcerative Colitis

Ulcerative colitis may be difficult to differentiate from gastrointestinal milk allergy because it often improves on a milk-free diet. In fact, milk allergy has been proposed as having a role in some cases of ulcerative colitis, as suggested by the presence of high titers of antibodies to milk.[30-32] Nevertheless, well-established ulcerative colitis rarely clears completely on simple elimination of milk from the diet. Sigmoidoscopy and barium enema studies are important diagnostic tools.

Gastroenteritis

Diarrhea caused by viral or bacterial gastroenteritis or toxins in contaminated food is more commonly encountered beyond infancy than is gastrointestinal milk allergy. A history of exposure or of similar symptoms in family members, as well as laboratory identification of the offending agent, should support the diagnosis. Infants recovering from gastroenteritis of diverse causes may remain intolerant to milk for several days or weeks because of a secondary lactase deficiency.[33-36]

Intestinal Obstruction

The symptoms of hypertrophic pyloric stenosis, malrotation, intussusception, or other congenital or acquired surgical problems of the gastrointestinal tract may mimic milk allergy. Because these conditions often lead to rapid clinical deterioration, their early recognition and prompt management are of utmost importance.

Intestinal Parasites

Parasitic infestations, particularly in the tropics, are a common cause of gastrointestinal disturbances, malabsorption, failure to thrive, eosinophilia, and elevated serum level of IgE, all of which are common in gastrointestinal allergy to cow's milk. The following parasites should be considered in children suspected of having milk allergy.

Giardia lamblia, which may be demonstrated in the stools or duodenal aspirate.

Strongyloides stercoralis, which has characteristic rhabditiform larvae that may be found in the stools or in a small-bowel suction biopsy.

Capillaria philippinensis, which is present only in the Philippines and can be diagnosed by the characteristic ova in the stools.

Coccidia, which is difficult to diagnose; may be detected in the stools by the zinc phosphate flotation method or in a small-bowel biopsy.

Intestinal Lymphangiectasia

Lymphangiectasia of the small intestine is often associated with chylothorax, chylous ascites, or lymphedema in distal parts of the body. Characteristics of the disease are a decreased absorption of fat and exudation of lymph with loss of protein and lymphocytes into the gut. The patient may have steatorrhea, hypogammaglobulinemia, and impaired cell-mediated immunity. Diagnosis is by intestinal biopsy or lymphangiography.

Abetalipoproteinemia

Abetalipoproteinemia, a defect in the synthesis of beta-lipoprotein, is a rare disorder that causes steatorrhea during early infancy and may be recognized by acanthosis of the erythrocytes and an abnormal electrophoretic pattern of lipoproteins. Ataxic neuropathy develops in later childhood, and retinitis pigmentosa appears in early adulthood. Cholesterol, phospholipid, and triglyceride levels are reduced, and beta-lipoproteins are absent. Microscopic examination of the intestinal mucosa shows fat globules in the epithelial cells.

Immunodeficiency Diseases

Either B-cell or T-cell dysfunction may be associated with chronic diarrhea. It is most prominent among patients with defective cell-mediated immunity and particularly in infants with severe combined immunodeficiency. It is less common in the acquired types of hypogammaglobulinemia and relatively rare in congenital sex-linked hypogammaglobulinemia. The diarrhea in any of these conditions may be a result of infestation with *Giardia lamblia* or of excessive growth of bacteria or viruses. Bloody diarrhea is common in children with Wiskott-Aldrich syndrome and is probably secondary to both immune dysfunction and thrombocytopenia. A variety of gastrointestinal disorders, including celiac disease and cow's milk allergy, occur with increased frequency in subjects with an isolated deficiency of serum and secretory IgA.

Whipple's Disease

Whipple's disease, or intestinal lipodystrophy, is a rare disorder that occurs mainly in adult males. It may be manifested by arthritis or arthralgia, hyperpigmentation of the skin, abdominal pain, diarrhea, and malabsorption. The symptoms ameliorate with antibiotic therapy, suggesting a microbiologic cause. The intestinal biopsy specimen stained with periodic acid-Schiff reveals positive staining of small bodies within the intestinal macrophages.

Wolman's Disease

Wolman's disease is a rare familial form of lipidosis that becomes evident in the early weeks of life with gastrointestinal symptoms such as vomiting, diarrhea, abdominal distention, and hepatosplenomegaly. There is vacuolization of the lymphocytes, and a small-bowel biopsy specimen shows lipid vacuoles in the histiocytes. Adrenal calcification is a common finding. Death usually occurs within a few months.

Hereditary Angioedema

Herditary angioedema, a nonallergic condition caused by a deficiency or malfunction of C1 esterase inhibitor, is often manifested as episodes of recurrent acute abdominal pain, vomiting, or diarrhea. Episodes of edema of extremities may be precipitated by trauma or temperature extremes. Emotional stress can precipitate attacks in some subjects, as can the ingestion of allergens in food-allergic subjects. If the disorder is not recognized, death from acute laryngeal edema may result. The diagnosis is established by measuring the serum C1 esterase inhibitor activity.

Urologic Problems

Urinary tract infections and urologic anomalies may present, especially during infancy, with vomiting, abdominal pain, irritability, poor feeding, or failure to thrive. Unless the condition is recognized early, renal damage may be irreversible. Microscopic examination of a clean sample of urine, urine culture, and radiographic studies are needed to establish the diagnosis.

Abdominal Epilepsy

An abdominal "epilepsy-equivalent" is an uncommon condition that usually affects older children before puberty. The child complains of recurrent gastrointestial upset, mainly abdominal pain, nausea, and vomiting. Routine evaluation fails to reveal a cause. To make the diagnosis, some physicians rely on the electroencephalogram, but it may not show abnormal findings in every patient. Other causes must be excluded as far as possible, and if response to anticonvulsants is dramatic and reproducible, a presumptive diagnosis of abdominal epilepsy is justified.

Lead Poisoning

Gastrointestinal absorption of lead in children may result in chronic abdominal pain (lead colic), vomiting, anorexia, irritability, and anemia. A flat x-ray film of the abdomen may reveal radiopaque flecks in the intestine, indicating recent ingestion of the lead-containing material. The diagnosis depends on the determination of blood lead levels, free-erythrocyte protoporphyrin, and urinary coproporphyrin.

Psychogenic Abdominal Pain

Children frequently complain of recurrent abdominal pain without a detectable organic cause. The pain is usually localized to the periumbilical or epigastric region. A psychologic cause may be suggested by a tactfully taken history that

Differential Diagnosis

may reveal a relationship between the onset of pain and certain situational or emotional factors. Skilled psychologic and social evaluations may be needed to reveal the underlying cause.

RESPIRATORY DISORDERS

Nonallergic Rhinitis

INFECTIOUS RHINITIS

Rhinitis caused by upper respiratory infection is often associated with general malaise, sore throat, fever, mucopurulent nasal discharge, and swollen reddish turbinates. Concurrent similar illness in the family members or other contacts is common. Sneezing, itching, and nasal eosinophilia are usually minimal, as is the response to antihistamines.

VASOMOTOR RHINITIS

Vasomotor rhinitis is believed to be an exaggerated response of the autonomic nervous system to sudden changes in temperature, inhaled irritants, or alcohol ingestion. The condition occurs mainly in adults, and symptoms are similar to allergic rhinitis. Nasal blockage and watery rhinorrhea occur suddenly and fade within a few hours. Nasal eosinophilia is minimal, and the response to antihistamines is not dramatic.

Wheezing

In the differential diagnosis, in addition to asthma, a large number of causes of acute and chronic wheezing must be considered. Detailing the features of each cause is beyond the scope of this chapter. A partial list of conditions causing wheezing in a child is given below:

Bronchial asthma
Respiratory infection
   Bronchiolitis
   Acute laryngotracheobronchitis
   Bronchitis
   Pneumonia
Foreign body in trachea or bronchi
Congenital anomalies of trachea or bronchi
Vascular rings
Cystic fibrosis
α_1-antitrypsin deficiency
Hypersensitivity pneumonitis; inhaled organic dusts or chemicals

Bronchopulmonary aspergillosis
Pulmonary hemosiderosis
Left-sided heart failure; increased pulmonary venous pressure
Mediastinal masses
  Lymph nodes
  Enlarged thymus
  Retrosternal goiter
  Cysts

Aspiration

The role of aspiration in chronic pulmonary disease has been recently appreciated through several studies.[37-39] Aspiration may result from an incoordination in the swallowing mechanism, an esophageal or tracheal anomaly, or gastroesophageal reflux. In the latter condition, aspiration of gastric contents is facilitated by recumbency. Aspiration should be considered as a possible primary or contributory factor in all patients with chronic pulmonary symptoms or recurrent pneumonias, particularly if the symptoms were at any time precipitated by lying down. Evaluation should include a careful neurologic examination, radiographic studies, esophageal manometry, and esophageal pH studies (Tuttle test).

Pulmonary Hemosiderosis

Pulmonary hemosiderosis signifies a diffuse interstitial bleeding in the lungs resulting in an abnormal accumulation of hemosiderin (an iron hydroxide-protein complex) in the lungs. A simple classification[40] of the disease is presented below:

Primary
  Isolated
  With cardiac or pancreatic involvement
  With glomerulonephritis (Goodpasture's disease)
  With cow's milk allergy
Secondary to
  Cardiac disease
    Mitral stenosis
    Left ventricular failure
    Cor triatriatum
  Connective tissue disease
    Polyarteritis nodosa
    Systemic lupus erythematosus
    Rheumatoid lung disease

Purpuric disease
   Anaphylactoid purpura (Henoch-Schönlein)
   Thrombocytopenic purpura

In children, primary pulmonary hemosiderosis is more common than the secondary varieties. In adults, on the other hand, the disorder is frequently secondary to a cardiac disease causing pulmonary venous hypertension, or to a connective tissue disease causing vasculitis.

DERMATOLOGIC DISORDERS

Dermatologic manifestations of milk allergy, particularly in young children, may be confused with many nonallergic conditions. A few conditions, in particular, deserve brief mention here:

Irritation Rashes

Dermal eruptions in the diaper area are frequently secondary to urinary ammoniacal irritation. Perianal rashes associated with diarrheal stools may similarly be secondary to irritation and maceration. Intertrigo may result from heat and sweat retention along skin folds, causing hyperemia, maceration, and an eczematous appearance.

Seborrheic Dermatitis

Seborrheic dermatitis is often difficult to differentiate clearly from atopic dermatitis, particularly during early infancy. Generally, the infant with seborrhea is not as irritable or uncomfortable from pruritus as is the infant with atopic dermatitis. In one study, allergy to cow's milk was thought to play a major causative role in a high proportion of infants with seborrhea.[41]

Leiner's Disease

Leiner's disease, also called erythroderma desquamativa, is usually manifest in the first few weeks of life as a generalized seborrheic dermatitis, which may be accompanied by severe diarrhea and susceptibility to infection. In some patients, C5a activity has been defective.[42]

Acrodermatitis Enteropathica

In acrodermatitis enteropathica, a vesiculobullous eczematous eruption beginning in the perianal area is accompanied by hair loss and severe diarrhea. The disease was formerly almost universally fatal during early infancy. Recent studies have shown that many cases are caused by zinc deficiency and that successful treatment is possible by dietary supplementation with zinc.[43] Since the zinc content in cow's milk is lower than in human milk, zinc deficiency would be enhanced in the presence of cow's milk-induced malabsorption. In such infants, it is prudent as well to restrict the intake of cow's milk and to ensure a well balanced diet.

Candidiasis

Cutaneous candidiasis usually involves the warm, moist, intertrigenous areas. The affected area typically has a well-demarcated severe erythema with scattered satellite lesions. The diagnosis is easily established by a microscopic examination of a KOH slide preparation from the lesion. The immunologic and endocrine status of children with chronic mucocutaneous candidiasis should be investigated.

Ichthyosis

Ichthyosiform dermatoses are characterized by generalized dryness, keratosis, and scaling of the skin. Inheritance may be autosomal dominant (ichthyosis vulgaris and epidermolytic hyperkeratosis), autosomal recessive (lamellar ichthyosis), or sex-linked (X-linked ichthyosis).

Insect Bites

Urticarial papular eruptions resulting from bites of various insects such as fleas, mites, lice, bedbugs, or mosquitoes are usually localized and evanescent. Nevertheless, the reaction may be extremely pruritic and lead to excoriations and infection. Some of the papules usually have a central dimple or puncture indicating the site of the insect bite and providing a valuable clue to the diagnosis. In sensitized subjects reactions may be severe.

REFERENCES

1. Collins-Williams C: Cow's milk allergy in infants and children. Int Arch Allergy 20:38–59, 1962
2. Speer F: Food allergy. Littleton, PSG Publishing Co, 1978, p 16
3. Federal Register 18:1077, 1953
4. Vickers HR, Bagratuni L, Alexander S: Dermatitis caused by penicillin in milk. Lancet 1:351–352, 1958
5. Borrie P, Barrett J: Dermatitis caused by penicillin in bulked milk supplies. Br Med J 2:1267, 1961

6. Wicher K, Reisman RE, Arbesman CE: Allergic reaction to penicillin present in milk. JAMA 208:143–145, 1969
7. Ament ME: Malabsorption syndromes in infancy and childhood. Part I. J Pediatr 81:685–697, 1972
8. Ament ME: Malabsorption syndromes in infancy and childhood. Part II. J Pediatr 81:867–884, 1972
9. Lockey SD: Reactions to hidden agents in foods, beverages and drugs. Ann Allergy 29:461–466, 1971
10. Michaelsson G, Juhlin L: Urticaria induced by preservatives and dye additives in foods and drugs. Br J Dermatol 88:525–532, 1973
11. Lebenthal E: Small intestinal disaccharidase deficiencies. Pediatr Clin North Am 22:757–766, 1975
12. Lloyd-Still JD: Chronic diarrhea of childhood and the misuse of elimination diets. J Pediatr 95:10–13, 1979
13. Lubos MC, Gerrard JW, Buchan DJ: Disaccharidase activities in milk-sensitive and celiac patients. J Pediatr 70:325–331, 1967
14. Liu H-Y, Tsao MU, Moore B, et al.: Bovine milk protein-induced intestinal malabsorption of lactose and fat in infants. Gastroenterology 54:27–34, 1968
15. Silver H, Douglas DM: Milk intolerance in infancy. Arch Dis Child 43:17–22, 1968
16. Sutton RE, Hamilton JR: Tolerance of young children with severe gastroenteritis to dietary lactose: A controlled study. Can Med Assoc J 99:980–982, 1968
17. Matsumura T, Kuroume T, Amada K: Close relationship between lactose intolerance and allergy to milk protein. J Asthma Res 9:13–19, 1971
18. Harrison M, Kilby A, Walker-Smith JA, et al.: Cow's milk protein intolerance: A possible association with gastroenteritis, lactose intolerance, and IgA deficiency. Br Med J 1:1501–1504, 1976
19. Poley JR, Bhatia M, Welsh JD: Disaccharidase deficiency in infants with cow's milk protein intolerance: Response to treatment. Digestion 17:97–107, 1978
20. Spies JR: New antigens in lactose (35546). Proc Soc Exp Biol Med 137:211–214, 1971
21. Katz AJ, Falchuk ZM: Current concepts in gluten sensitive enteropathy (celiac sprue). Pediatr Clin North Am 22:767–785, 1975
22. Heiner DC, Lahey ME, Wilson JF, et al.: Precipitins to antigens of wheat and cow's milk in celiac disease. J Pediatr 61:813–830, 1962
23. Gerrard JW, Heiner DC, Ives EJ, et al.: Milk allergy: Recognition, natural history and management. Clin Pediatr 2:634–641, 1963
24. Clein NW: Cow's milk allergy in infants. Pediatr Clin North Am 4:949–962, 1954
25. Gryboski JD, Katz J, Reynolds D, et al.: Gluten intolerance following cow's milk sensitivity: Two cases with coproantibodies to milk and wheat proteins. Ann Allergy 26:33–39, 1968
26. Kuitunen P, Visakorpi JK, Savilahti E, et al.: Malabsorption syndrome with cow's milk intolerance. Arch Dis Child 50:351–356, 1975
27. Visakorpi JK, Immonen P: Intolerance to cow's milk and wheat gluten in the primary malabsorption syndrome in infancy. Acta Paediatr Scand 56:49–56, 1967
28. Shwachman H: Gastrointestinal manifestations of cystic fibrosis. Pediatr Clin North Am 22:787–805, 1975
29. Shwachman H, Diamond LK, Oski FA, et al.: The syndrome of pancreatic insufficiency and bone marrow dysfunction. J Pediatr 65:645–663, 1964
30. Davidson L: Milk proteins in ulcerative colitis. Br Med J 2:1358, 1961
31. Taylor KB, Truelove SC: Circulating antibodies to milk proteins in ulcerative colitis. Br Med J 2:924–929, 1961
32. Dudek B, Spiro HH, Thayer WR: A study of ulcerative colitis and circulating antibodies to milk proteins. Gastroenterology 49:544–547, 1965

33. Sheehy TW, Artenstein MS, Green RW: Small intestinal mucosa in certain viral diseases. JAMA 190:1023–1028, 1964
34. Lifshitz R, Coello-Ramirez P, Gutierriz-Topete G, et al.: Carbohydrate intolerance in infants with diarrhea. J Pediatr 79:760–767, 1971
35. Leake RD, Schroeder KC, Benton DA, et al.: Soy-based formula in the treatment of infantile diarrhea. Am J Dis Child 127:374–376, 1974
36. Iyngkaran N, Davis K, Robinson MJ et al.: Cow's milk protein-sensitive enteropathy: An important contributing cause of secondary sugar intolerance in young infants with acute infective enteritis. Arch Dis Child 54:39–43, 1979
37. Danus O, Casar C, Larrain A, et al.: Esophageal reflux: An unrecognized cause of recurrent obstructive bronchitis in children. J Pediatr 89:220–224, 1976
38. Euler AR, Byrne WJ, Ament ME, et al.: Recurrent pulmonary disease in children: A complication of gastroesophageal reflux. Pediatrics 63:47–51, 1979
39. Shapiro GG, Christie DL: Gastroesophagel reflux in steroid-dependent asthmatic youths. Pediatrics 63:207–212, 1979
40. Heiner DC: Pulmonary hemosiderosis, in Kendig EL, Jr, Chernick V (eds): Disorders of the Respiratory Tract in Children. Philadelphia, Saunders, 1977, pp 538–552
41. Eppig JJ: Seborrhea capitis in infants: A clinical experience in allergy therapy. Ann Allergy 29:323–324, 1971
42. Miller ME, Koblenzer PJ: Leiner's disease and deficiency of C5. J Pediatr 80:879–881, 1972
43. Moynahan EJ: Acrodermatitis enteropathica: A lethal inherited human zinc disorder. Lancet 2:399–400, 1974

8
Management

An outline for the management of milk allergy is presented below:[1]

    Dietary Management
        Elimination of cow's milk
        Elimination of other offending allergens
        Provide cow's milk substitutes
    Pharmacologic Agents For
        Symptomatic therapy
        Treatment of sequelae
        Prophylactic medication
    Hyposensitization (unproved)

DIETARY MANAGEMENT

The basic treatment of food allergies is to eliminate the offending allergen from the diet. Obviously, both recognizing and avoiding responsible allergens are essential for obtaining optimal results.

Milk Elimination

Once the diagnosis of milk allergy has been established, a program designed to ensure the highest attainable degree of avoiding cow's milk should be instituted. Initially, strict avoidance of milk and all milk products is recommended. Later, careful challenge-testing may indicate that symptoms occur after the intake of certain forms of milk or of critical quantities but not after consumption of other milk-containing preparations (e.g., heated milk) or of small quantities taken at widely spaced intervals.

In young infants, milk in the diet can be strictly avoided relatively easily. In the first 6 months of life, the infant usually can be given a single milk substitute. Solid nonmilk-containing foods can then be introduced into the infant's diet according to plans made jointly by the parents and the physician. The conservative approach of avoiding common allergenic foods such as eggs, or foods to which other family members have been allergic, until about 6 months of age is preferred. New foods are introduced one at a time at about 1-week intervals when the infant is not suffering from an illness or having allergic symptoms. In this way, additional food intolerances are most readily recognized.

In older children and adults, cow's milk is often difficult to eliminate completely, because milk is incorporated into many common items in the daily diet. Patients often must limit themselves to fruits, vegetables, and foods prepared at home from milk-free ingredients.

In addition to the obvious milk products such as butter and cream, a large number of milk-containing foods are sold by commercial suppliers. Some common items are listed below:

Butter	Ice cream
Buttermilk	Luncheon meats
Biscuits (most)	Macaroni
Bread (most)	Malted milk
Cakes	Meatloaf
Candies (many)	Milk shakes
Caramels	Sherbet
Cereals (some)	Noodles
Cheese	Nougat
Chocolate	Ovaltine
Chowder	Puddings
Crackers	Rolls
Cream soups	Sauces
Creamed vegetables	Sausages
Cocomalt	Sour milk
Custards	Waffles
Frankfurters	Yogurt

Ordinary margarine contains small quantities of cow's milk proteins, whereas kosher oleomargarine (pure vegetable oil) contains no milk. Milk powder is commonly added to frankfurters, luncheon meats, and other processed meats. The labels of all commercially prepared foods must be checked. In the United States, the Food and Drug Administration now requests that food manufacturers list on the label all ingredients of prepared foods. Unfortunately, this regulation is not fully enforced and is not thoroughly accepted by the food industry. Many marketed food preparations are still inadequately labeled.

Fortunately, few milk-sensitive patients are so senstive that minute hidden quantities of milk will result in severe reactions. Many patients can tolerate small quantities of milk with minimal or no symptoms. Indeed, in such patients, complete avoidance of milk at times may impose an unnecessary social or psychologic burden. The occasional intake of small well-tolerated quantities of milk-containing foods may be of more value than harm to some patients, particularly older children and adolescents who are concerned with social events such as birthday parties or dating. The physician should show discretion and encourage the exercise of wisdom in such circumstances.

DURATION OF MILK ELIMINATION

The duration of milk sensitivity may vary from several months to several years, or it may be lifelong (see Chap. 9). Because the maturation of the gastrointestinal tract may play an important role, we generally suggest that a milk-sensitive infant not be fed cow's milk for about 6 months or until 1 year of age. Then, to determine whether the patient is still sensitive to milk, the physician gives him an oral milk challenge, under appropriate supervision. If symptoms occur, a strict milk-elimination diet should be reinstituted. The diet is interrupted every 6 to 18 months by a deliberate oral challenge. In some instances, the persistence or disappearance of sensitivity is discovered by the patient himself, through accidental or willful ingestion of milk. Whenever a high degree of sensitivity has been manifest in the past, challenges should be made under the direct supervision of a physician so that appropriate emergency treatment can be given if necessary.

Elimination of Other Offending Allergens

In many milk-sensitive subjects, elimination of cow's milk alone fails to result in total disappearance of symptoms. Often these persons also are sensitive to inhalants or other foods. Frequently, associated food allergens are soybean, orange, egg, wheat, rice, oats, tomato, pork, beef, and chicken.[2,3] Allergens often have an additive or synergistic effect. In some milk-sensitive patients, the control of a concomitant ingestant or inhalant allergy may result in better tolerance to cow's milk.[4]

Occasionally, patients sensitive to bovine-serum constituents that are present in cow's milk, such as albumin or gamma globulin, develop symptoms on eating incompletely cooked beef. Also, in rare instances, contact with cows themselves or cow hair products such as mohair or felt padding, or inhalation of cow dander, may aggravate respiratory allergies caused by milk ingestion.[5]

Milk Substitutes

Infants and young children sensitive to cow's milk need a suitable substitute formula, whereas for older children and adults, simple fruits, vegetables, and meats are adequate substitutes. Listed below are milk substitutes commonly available in most countries:

Soybean formulas
Heat-treated cow's milk
Protein hydrolysates
Elemental diets
Goat's milk
Meat base formula
Vegetable formulas
Homemade preparations
Human milk

Generally speaking, an optimal milk substitute should meet the following requirements:

1. *High nutritional value.* For optimal growth of the greatest number of infants, a preparation must contain protein, fat, and carbohydrate in quantities roughly similar to those in human milk, together with an adequate supplement of essential vitamins and minerals.
2. *Low allergenicity.* This can be demonstrated by both immunologic and clinical studies.
3. *Simplicity of preparation.* Formulas for newborn infants should be easy to prepare in liquid form in proper concentration and with optimal osmolality.
4. *Acceptable taste and odor.* This will ensure an adequate intake.
5. *Ready availability and reasonable price.* This is essential for marketed preparations because expensive or difficult-to-find foods discourage compliance with the milk-free diet.

SOYBEAN FORMULAS

The first report on soybean "milk" in infant feeding was probably in 1909 by Ruhräh,[6] who substituted it for cow's milk in gastrointestinal disorders. In 1917, Osborne and Mendel[7] reported that soybean was nutritionally adequate for the normal growth of infants. In 1929, Hill recommended the use of a soybean preparation for feeding infants with cow's milk idiosyncrasy.[8,9] By the 1950s, formulas utilizing soy flour were widely available in the United States. Experiments involving dual-ingestion passive-transfer testing[10] and guinea-pig anaphylaxis[11] showed a low allergenicity of heat-treated soy protein. As with heat-treated cow's milk, the antigenicity of heat-processed soy protein isolate, as tested by immunoelectrophoretic and gel-diffusion techniques, was lower than the antigenicity of unheated soy flour formula.[12] At present, nearly all soy flour formulas have been replaced by water-soluble soy protein isolate formulas.

Soybean isolate formulas are now widely available at a reasonable cost in most countries. They are well accepted by most children, and their nutritional value is comparable to that of cow's milk formulas.[13-16] They can also replace cow's milk in the preparation of a great variety of foods, including beverages, ice cream, cookies, main dishes, and desserts (see Appendix A for recipes).

Like other proteins, soy protein is antigenic in man,[17] and clinical hypersensitivity is not uncommon.[2,3,18-22] Probably about one fourth of milk-sensitive patients become allergic to soy protein after its prolonged ingestion.[2,3] The symptoms may be similar to or different from those caused by milk allergy.

Ament and Rubin[23] observed complete loss of the jejunal villi and flattening of the mucosa, similar to that seen in celiac disease, in a 6-week-old infant who developed severe gastrointestinal symptoms within 24 hours of ingesting soy formula. After the infant's recovery, the symptoms and histologic changes were reproduced by oral challenge with soy protein but not with soy lecithin, gluten, or cow's milk.

Diarrhea from soy formula, however, may not always be caused by hypersensitivity; it may be secondary to fermentation of the indigestible carbohydrate stachyose.[24] It occurs less frequently with the use of soy protein isolate than with soy flour formulas. Soy-induced diarrhea is often diminished on using a half-strength formula for a few days or using a preparation with glucose as the only carbohydrate. A simple constipating mixture added to the bottle may be helpful. If these measures do not help, a change should be made to another milk substitute.

Some soybean formulas (such as Neo-Mull-Soy—Syntex) have a low chloride content. Infants who are fed such a formula may occasionally develop hypochloremic alkalosis.[24a] In these instances, an adequate dietary supplement of chloride must be insured.

The composition of commonly available soy formulas is presented in Appendix B, Table 5. The caloric content is almost the same in various preparations (20 Kcal/oz or 0.67 Kcal/ml), but the distribution of calories between protein, fat, and carbohydrate varies somewhat. In most preparations, the fat is in the form of soy oil and the carbohydrate largely in the form of sucrose.

HEAT-TREATED COW'S MILK

As mentioned in Chapter 4, heat treatment of cow's milk proteins results in denaturation of the bovine serum albumin and immunoglobulin. Alpha-lactalbumin is slightly less heat-labile, whereas beta-lactoglobulin is moderately heat-stable and casein is highly heat-stable.

Boiled or evaporated milks may be well tolerated by patients sensitive solely to the heat-labile protein fractions but poorly tolerated by patients sensitive to casein. A patient who is not highly sensitive to heat-stable constituents of cow's milk and has been asymptomatic for a few months on a milk-free diet may be able to tolerate evaporated or boiled milk.[25-27] The cost of feeding evaporated milk to infants is usually less than that of feeding a ready-to-use milk formula. The composition of reconstituted evaporated formula is similar to that of the ready-to-feed milk formulas (Appendix B, Table 4).

PROTEIN HYDROLYSATES

Special formulas are available in which protein is provided as an enzymatic hydrolysate of bovine casein. The digested casein is usually subjected to filtration procedures that separate and remove the large undigested protein molecules from the amino acids and smaller polypeptides.

Hydrolysates are more readily assimilated and considerably less allergenic than the native protein molecules. Formulas containing such hydrolysates are nutritionally adequate and well tolerated by most children.[24,28-30]

Examples of these formulas are Nutramigen and Pregestimil (Mead-Johnson) (Appendix B, Table 5). Both of these preparations contain corn oil and are devoid of lactose. Pregestimil contains medium-chain triglycerides, which are easily absorbed through the portal system. It, therefore, is useful not only in milk allergies but also in conditions associated with abnormalities in bile secretion or in intestinal lymphatics. Nutramigen is a satisfactory formula for most milk-sensitive infants and is less expensive than Pregestimil. It also has a lower osmolarity than Pregestimil (397 vs 449 mOsm/liter).

ELEMENTAL DIETS

In elemental diets, protein is replaced by synthetic amino acids. The diets contain no protein from animal or plant sources. An example of such a diet is Vivonex (Eaton), which is composed of L–amino acids, glucose, safflower oil, electrolytes, and vitamins (Appendix B, Table 5). It is nutritionally adequate in most instances, and children generally gain weight well on it unless they do not accept its taste. Vivonex Standard provides 1 Kcal/ml; 90.2 percent from glucose, 8.5 percent from amino acids, and 1.3 percent from safflower oil, and it has an osmolarity of 500 mOsm per liter.

Elemental diets are residue-free and have been successfully used in a variety of severe gastrointestinal diseases, both in infants[31-33] and in adults.[34] Sera of rabbits immunized with Vivonex did not develop antibodies demonstrable by precipitin or passive cutaneous anaphylaxis reactions, indicating a low immunogenicity of the preparation.[35]

Vivonex is often of value in milk-sensitive patients who do not tolerate other milk substitutes or as an initial diet in patients with severe multiple food intolerances. It is available in several flavors; however, the unflavored form, which is usually well accepted by infants though less well accepted by older children, is preferred because its use avoids possible untoward reactions from flavoring additives.

GOAT'S MILK

The composition of goat's milk resembles that of cow's milk (Appendix B, Table 4). Immunologic cross-reactivity exists between many goat- and cow-milk proteins, especially the caseins, beta-lactoglobulin and alpha-lactalbumin.[24,36-38] Perhaps one-third of infants who are sensitive to cow's milk are able to tolerate goat's milk. Also goat's milk is not widely available and, unless supplemented with folic acid, its use ocasionally results in the development of megaloblastic anemia. With the availability of a wide variety of more acceptable milk substitutes, goat's milk is now seldom recommended.

MEAT-BASE FORMULA

A meat-base formula has been commercially available (Meat Base Formula — Gerber). Its protein source is beef heart, and it does not contain lactose. It is nutritionally adequate (Appendix B, Table 5) and usually well accepted by children. It is worth trying in milk-sensitive infants who do not tolerate other substitues.[29]

VEGETABLE DIETS

Diet preparations are being developed from vegetables, fruits, legumes, and cereals.[39,40] Poi, a paste made of taro *(Colcasia esculenta),* has also been suggested as a hypoallergenic diet.[41] These diets may be particularly useful in some children with stubborn multiple-food sensitivities. Until thoroughly documented and standardized, however, their nutritional adequacy as a complete diet is uncertain, even with added vitamins. Vegetables frequently are lacking in the proteins needed for optimal growth.

HOMEMADE PREPARATIONS

Beyond early infancy, the milk-sensitive subject is likely to be frequently exposed to foods containing various quantities of milk, as well as other potentially allergenic substances. Manufactured foods frequently contain milk constitutents or other ingredients that are either listed on the label in small print or not listed at all. Information on ingredients is particularly important to patients who may also be sensitive to preservatives, coloring or flavoring agents, or trace contaminants. It is both safer and more economical to restrict the diet of certain allergic persons to homemade foods prepared from simple ingredients. In many instaces, consultation with a dietician greatly helps the family that must plan a nutritionally adequate diet. A variety of milk-free recipes are provided in Appendix A.

HUMAN MILK

In rare instances, a young infant does not tolerate or accept any of the commercially available infant formulas. For such infants, human breast milk may be the only suitable food for several months. Unfortunately, human milk banks still are not widely available and the supply of human milk is severely limited.

PHARMACOLOGIC AGENTS

In the management of food allergy, pharmacologic agents may help prevent and control symptoms. Unless the offending allergens are avoided, however, the response to drug therapy is usually suboptimal.

Symptomatic Therapy

The drug of choice for the control of symptoms varies from one person to another and depends to some degree on the type and chronicity of symptoms. Acute reactions are best treated with epinephrine, aminophylline, or antihistamines, or combinations of these drugs. In acute anaphylaxis, all three medications should be given parenterally, and the airway must be maintained, intravenous fluids given, and additional drugs such as vasopressor amines may be needed. Rhinitis and itching often respond to oral antihistamines. In severe atopic dermatitis, topical and sometimes systemic corticosteroid therapy may be especially effective. Oral corticosteroids and antihistamines can speed recovery from milk-induced gastroenteropathy.

Treatment of Sequelae

In patients with prolonged vomiting or diarrhea, the correction of fluid loss and electrolyte imbalance is most important. If the patient does not tolerate oral feedings after a week or so of receiving parenteral fluids, intravenous alimentation may be required, sometimes for prolonged periods, until the intestinal mucosa has regenerated and matured to the point that oral feedings of a hypoallergenic formula can be tolerated. Concurrent infections should be treated with appropriate antibiotics. Nutrition and growth should be carefully monitored until full recovery, which in some instances may not be attained for months or years. Correction of anemia often requires iron therapy, and occasionally vitamin C and folic acid as well.

Prophylactic Medication

When the offending food allergen cannot be strictly avoided, symptoms may persist or recur. In such instances, drugs used judiciously may prevent or significantly reduce the effects of allergen ingestion.

ANTIHISTAMINES

These may be given orally 20 to 60 minutes before an anticipated exposure to the offending food on occasions such as a birthday party when eating a small amount of ice cream, for example, might be psychologically important to the child. In other circumstances, such as when an infant tolerates cow's milk formulas poorly and also has difficulty with milk-substitute formulas, giving a small dose of an antihistamine with each feeding may permit the infant to thrive. Often the use of one-half and sometimes one-quarter of the usual therapeutic dose effectively prevents symptoms.

INHIBITORS OF PROSTAGLANDIN SYNTHESIS

These may be worth trying if the level of prostaglandin E_2 or $F_2\alpha$ is increased in the plasma or in secretions of the shock organ. In one study[42] the development of untoward reactions was prevented in 5 out of 6 food-sensitive patients by the intake of aspirin, indomethacin, or ibuprofen before challenge with the food.

DISODIUM CROMOGLYCATE (CROMOLYN).

Administered orally, cromolyn has shown promising results in several studies on patients with allergies to cow's milk or to other foods.[43-51] The drug seems to be most effective in controlling gastrointestinal symptoms, but symptoms in other systems are also ameliorated in varying degrees.

The drug may be taken in a capsule that dissolves easily in the stomach or as a fresh aqueous solution, in which it has a bland taste. In exquisitely-sensitive patients, the aqueous form may be used to rinse the mouth before being swallowed. In this way, reactions that may result from antigen absorption through the oral mucosa may be prevented. The dosage and frequency of administration vary from patient to patient, depending more on the degree of exposure to the offending food and the degree of hypersensitivity than on the patient's age. Best results are obtained when the drug is taken 20 to 60 minutes before exposure to the food allergen. The protective effect may last for 3 or 4 hours. Infrequently, it may be given before, and for 24 to 48 hours after, an anticipated exposure, or on a continuous, 4 times daily, basis in patients with frequent symptoms. In the average patient, a dose between 50 and 200 mg is optimal. Some patients do well on a dose as low as 25 mg, whereas others may need up to 800 mg per dose. The preparation of cromolyn used for inhalation in bronchial asthma contains lactose, which may also contain traces of bovine milk proteins, and therefore its oral intake may aggravate the symptoms of milk allergy especially in the presence of lactase deficiency.

The action of oral cromolyn on the gastrointestinal tract is probably similar to the action of inhaled cromolyn on the bronchial tree, i.e., inhibition of the release of chemical mediators from sensitized mast cells. The drug is minimally absorbed through the gastrointestinal mucosa.[52]

How orally administered cromolyn prevents nongastrointestinal symptoms of food allergy is not clear. Possibly, such symptoms are caused by chemical mediators that are released from the gastrointestinal tract, reach the circulation, and thus produce symptoms in distant organs. The drug has been administered to patients of various ages, including young infants, and most investigators have not noticed significant side-effects during its use. Gerrard,[51] however, gave 80 patients, with various adverse reactions to foods, 50 to 100 mg cromolyn orally 4 times a day, and 14 patients (18 percent) complained of adverse effects: headache in 6; urticaria in 3; abdominal pain in 2; diarrhea in 2; rhinorrhea in 1; vomiting in 1; insomnia in 1; and depression in 1. More studies are needed to define the adverse effects of prolonged usage of the drug. Further studies are also needed to learn how effective oral cromoly is in normalizing the gastrointestinal mucosa. Possibly mucosal damage permits the offending allergen to be absorbed in abnormal quantities, which may produce adverse reactions in remote shock organs. In this regard, Esteban et al[47] noted that two infants developed respiratory allergies despite their intake of oral cromolyn regularly for several months to control gastrointestinal food allergies. In a study[53] on patients with food-induced asthma, oral doses of 200 mg of cromolyn 4 times a day for a week or a single dose of 1 gm 30 minutes before oral challenge with the offending food could not prevent the development of bronchospasm.

At the present time, unrestricted ingestion of food allergens under cover of long-term oral cromolyn administration is not recommended. Rather, the use of oral cromolyn should be restricted to instances in which complete elimination of the offending food or foods cannot be achieved.

HYPOSENSITIZATION

Hyposensitization with food allergens, including milk, has been tried through both oral and injection routes but neither has gained significant acceptance. Successful hyposensitization against foods has been shown in only few instances. The few scattered reports in the literature are not convincing enough for the procedure to be recommended for the routine management of food allergy.[54]

Oral Hyposensitization

Finkelstein,[55] and later others,[56-59] reported oral hyposensitization with cow's milk as early as 1905. In each of these reports, however, the number of patients was too small to permit a scientifically sound conclusion.

The procedure usually consisted of giving drop quantities of diluted milk, increased in amount and strength every day according to the tolerance of the individual patient. When the maximum tolerable dose was reached, it was given daily. An increase in the dose was tried every few weeks until the desired level of intake was reached.

Studies on experimental animals have shown that repeated oral administration of certain antigens is an efficient method for the induction of immunologic unresponsiveness.[60-63] In man, however, the procedure has not been subjected to a well-controlled study on an adequate scale, and the supposed underlying immunologic mechanisms have not been elucidated.

Injection Hyposensitization

This type of hyposensitization for food allergy has received even less acceptance by most allergists, although subcutaneous injection of food extracts has been mentioned in the literature.[64,65] In one report,[66] the efficacy of the procedure was claimed to be enhanced by using "enzyme-potentiated extracts" prepared through a certain formulation of beta-glucuronidase, 1, 3, cyclohexane diol, protamine hyaluronidase, chondroitin sulfate, and buffer. Careful double-blind experiments have not confirmed the efficacy of injection hyposensitization for food allergy. A few practitioners have enthusiastically endorsed and are regularly using the subcutaneous or intracutaneous injection of food extracts for "desensitization" and for "neutralization" of ongoing or provoked symptoms. Although we do not consider it prudent to condemn such practices outright or to have a closed mind regarding their potential value, we believe it is important to develop such procedures carefully and in the spirit of scientific inquiry. Claims of success should be made with circumspection and with due consideration for placebo effect. Every effort should be made to provide a theoretical basis for observed successes that can be subjected to objective laboratory investigation by competent workers. Logically, if such a phenomenon as "neutralization" by allergen of ongoing symptoms exists, it must depend on mechanisms that can be subjected to scientific inquiry. Until such investigation is accomplished, the watchword should be responsibility of claims and statements both by proponents and critics. At present we do not believe that sufficient evidence supports the efficacy of antigen injection therapy for food allergy; the procedure cannot be recommended for use by anyone except those who are making a serious attempt to determine its efficacy scientifically and to delineate the involved mechanisms.

Sublingual Hyposensitization

(And provocation-neutralization procedures)

These methods have proponents just as do food-allergen injection techniques. Most such proponents are honorable practitioners who use sublingual administration of food allergens in attempts to diagnose, prevent, and treat food allergy. The comments made above concerning food injections apply here as well. A careful, concerted effort designed to answer questions rather than to prove one's point of view seems in order.

REFERENCES

1. Bahna SL: Control of milk allergy: A challenge for physicians, mothers and industry. Ann Allergy 41:1–12, 1978
2. Gerrard JW, Lubos MC, Hardy LW, et al.: Milk allergy: Clinical picture and familial incidence. Can Med Assoc J 97:780–785, 1967

3. Gerrard JW, MacKenzie JWA, Goluboff N, et al.: Cow's milk allergy: Prevalence and manifestations in an unselected series of newborns. Acta Paediatr Scand Suppl 234:1–21, 1973
4. Goldstein GB, Heiner DC: Clinical and immunological perspectives in food sensitivity. J Allergy 46:270–291, 1970
5. Osvath P, Muranyi L, Endré L, et al.: Investigation of the cross reaction of cow's hair and milk antigen in bronchial provocation. Acta Allergol (Kbh) 27:355–363, 1972
6. Ruhräh J: The soybean in infant feeding: Preliminary report. Arch Pediatr 26:496–501, 1909
7. Osborne TH, Mendel LB: The use of soybean as food. J Biol Chem 32:369–387, 1917
8. Hill LW, Stuart HC: A soybean food preparation for feeding infants with milk idiosyncrasy. JAMA 93:985–987, 1929
9. Hill LW: Infantile eczema with a special reference to the use of a milk-free diet. JAMA 96:1277–1280, 1931
10. Ratner B, Untracht S, Crawford LV, et al.: Allergenicity of modified and processed foodstuffs. V. Soybean: Influence of heat on its allergenicity; use of soybean preparations as milk substitutes. Am J Dis Child 89:187–193, 1955
11. Ratner B, Crawford LV: Soybean: Anaphylactic properties. Ann Allergy 13:289–295, 1955
12. Crawford LV, Roane J, Triplett F, et al.: Immunologic studies on the legume family of foods. Ann Allergy 23:303–308, 1965
13. Glaser J, Johnstone DE: Soybean milk as a substitute for mammalian milk in early infancy; with special reference to prevention of allergy to cow's milk. Ann Allergy 10:433–439, 1952.
14. Kane S: Nutritional management of allergic reactions to cow's milk. Am Practitioner 8:65–69, 1957
15. Kay JL, Daeschner CW, Jr, Desmond MM: Evaluation of infants fed soybean and evaporated milk formulae from birth to three months: A comparison of weight, length, hemoglobin, hematocrit, and plasma biochemical values. Am J Dis Child 100:264–276, 1960
16. Graham GG, Placko RP, Morales E, et al.: Dietary protein quality in infants and children. VI. Isolated soy protein milk. Am J Dis Child 120:419–423, 1970
17. Eastham EJ, Lichauco T, Grady MI, et al.: Antigenicity of infant formulas: Role of immature intestine on protein permeability. J Pediatr 93:561–564, 1978
18. Mendoza J, Meyers J, Snyder R: Soybean sensitivity: A case report. Pediatrics 46:774–776, 1970
19. Powell GK: Enterocolitis in low-birth-weight infants associated with milk and soy protein intolerance. J Pediatr 88:840–844, 1976
20. Powell GK: Milk- and soy-induced enterocolitis of infancy: Clinical features and standardization of challenge. J Pediatr 93:553–560, 1978
21. Whitington PF, Gibson RG: Soy protein intolerance: Four patients with concomitant cow's milk intolerance. Pediatrics 59:730–732, 1977
22. Goel K, Lifshitz F, Kahn E, et al.: Monosaccharide intolerance and soy-protein hypersensitivity in an infant with diarrhea. J Pediatr 93:617–619, 1978
23. Ament ME, Rubin CE: Soy protein: Another cause of the flat intestinal lesion. Gastroenterology 62:227–234, 1972
24. Freier S, Kletter B: Milk allergy in infants and young children. Clin Pediatr 9:449–454, 1970
24a. Garin EH, Geary D, Richard GA: Soybean formula (Neo-Mull-Soy) metabolic alkalosis in infancy. J Pediatr 95:985–987, 1977
25. Collins-Williams C: Cow's milk allergy in infants and children. Int Arch Allergy 20:38–59, 1962
26. Goldman AS, Anderson DW, Jr, Sellers WA, et al.: Milk Allergy. I. Oral challenge with milk and isolated milk proteins in allergic children. Pediatrics 32:425–443, 1963
27. Frankland AW: Food allergies. R Soc Health J 90:243–247, 1970
28. Gryboski JD: Gastrointestinal milk allergy in infants. Pediatrics 40:354–362, 1967

29. Self TW, Herskovic T, Czapek E, et al.: Gastrointestinal protein allergy. JAMA 207:2393–2396, 1969
30. Freier S, Kletter B: Clinical and immunological aspects of milk protein intolerance. Aust Paediatr J 8:140–146, 1972
31. Stephens RV, Dury KD, Delucia FG, et al.: Use of an elemental diet in the nutritional management of catabolic disease in infants. Am J Surg 123:374–379, 1972
32. Sherman JO, Hamly CA, Khachadurian AK: Use of an oral elemental diet in infants with severe intractable diarrhea. J Pediatr 86:518–523, 1975
33. Nelson TL, Klein GL, Galant SP: Severe eosinophilic gastro-enteritis successfully treated with an elemental diet (Vivonex). J Allergy Clin Immunol 63:198, 1979
34. Rocchio MA, Cha CM, Haas KF, et al.: Use of chemically defined diets in the management of patients with acute inflammatory bowel disease. Am J Surg 127:469–475, 1974
35. Galant SP, Franz ML, Walker P, et al.: A potential diagnostic method for food allergy: Clinical application and immunogenicity evaluation of an elemental diet. Am J Clin Nutr 30:512–516, 1977
36. Saperstein S: Antigenicity of the whey proteins in evaporated cow's milk and whole goat's milk. Ann Allergy 18:765–773, 1960
37. Crawford LV, Grogan FT: Allergenicity of cow's milk proteins. IV. Relationship of goat's milk proteins as studied by serum-agar precipitation. J Pediatr 59:347–350, 1961
38. Lebenthal E, Laor J, Lewitus Z, et al.: Gastrointestinal protein loss in allergy to cow's milk β-lactoglobulin. Isr J Med Sci 6:506–510, 1970
39. Food and Nutrition Board, National Academy of Sciences: Vegetarian diets. Am J Clin Nutr 27:1095–1096, 1974
40. Vyhmeister IB, Register UD, Sonnenberg LM: Safe vegetarian diets for children. Pediatr Clin North Am 24:203, 1977
41. Glaser J, Lawrence RA, Harrison A, et al.: Poi: Its use as a food for normal, allergic and potentially allergic children. Ann Allergy 25:496–500, 1967
42. Buisseret PD, Youlten LJF, Heinzelmann DI, et al.: Prostaglandin-synthesis inhibitors in prophylaxis of food intolerance. Lancet 1:906–908, 1978
43. Freier S, Berger H: Disodium cromoglycate in gastrointestinal protein intolerance. Lancet 1:913–915, 1973
44. Kuzemko JA, Simpson KR: Treatment of allergy to cow's milk. Lancet 1:337–338, 1975
45. Basomba A, Campos A, Villalmanzo IG, et al.: The effect of sodium cromoglycate (SCG) in patients with food allergies. Acta Allergol (Kbh) Suppl 13:95–101, 1977
46. Dannaeus A, Foucard T, Johansson SGO: The effect of orally administered sodium cromoglycate on symptoms of food allergy. Clin Allergy 7:109–115, 1977
47. Esteban MM, Ojeda Casas JA, Laso Borrego MT, et al.: Oral disodium cromoglycate in food allergy: An open trial in four patients. Acta Allergol (Kbh) 32:413–425, 1977
48. Nizami RM, Lewin PK, Baboo MT: Oral cromolyn therapy in patients with food allergy: A preliminary report. Ann Allergy 39:102–105, 1977
49. Vaz GA, LKT, Gerrard JW: Oral cromoglycate in treatment of adverse reactions to foods. Lancet 1:1066–1068, 1978
50. Dannaeus A, Inganäs M, Johansson SGO, et al.: Intestinal uptake of ovalbumin in malabsorption and food allergy in relation to serum IgG antibody and orally administered sodium cromoglycate. Clin Allergy 9:263–270, 1979
50a. Kocoshis S, Grybosk JD: Use of cromolyn in combined gastrointestinal allergy. JAMA 242:1169–1173, 1979
51. Gerrard JW: Oral cromoglycate: Its value in the treatment of adverse reactions to foods. Ann Allergy 42:135–138, 1979
52. Walker WA, Bloch KJ, Davenport LM, et al.: Mechanism of antigen uptake from the small intestine. Ped Res 6:374, 1972

53. Harries MG, O'Brien IM, Burge PS, et al.: Effects of orally administered sodium cromoglycate in asthma and urticaria due to foods. Clin Allergy 8:423–427, 1978
54. Rowe AH: Food Allergy: Its Manifestations and Control, and the Elimination Diets, A Compendium. Springfield, Ill., Thomas, 1972, p 71
55. Finkelstein H: Kuhmilch als Ursache akuter Ernahrungstorungen bei Sauglingen. Monatsschr Kinderheilkd 4:65–72, 1905
56. Ratner B: The treatment of milk allergy and its basic principles. JAMA 105:934–939, 1935
57. Vendel S: Cow's milk idiosyncrasy in infants. Acta Paediatr Scand (Suppl 5) 35:3–37, 1948
58. Davies W: Cow's milk allergy in infancy. Arch Dis Child 33:265–268, 1958
59. Zalewski T, Foltanska H, Pulwarska E: Sensitization to cow milk. Ped Pol 46:159–164, 1971
60. Chase MW: Delayed sensitivity. Med Clin North Am 49:1613–1646, 1965
61. Thomas HD, Parrott MV: The induction of tolerance to a soluble protein antigen by oral administration. Immunology 27:631–639, 1974
62. David MF: Induction of unresponsiveness to particulate antigen by feeding. Ann Allergy 38:386, 1977
63. Hanson DG, Vaz NM, Maia LCS, et al.: Tolerance to proteins induced by feeding. Ann Allergy 38:386, 1977
64. Vaughan WT: Practice of Allergy. St. Louis, Mosby, 1939, p 337
65. Miller JB: A double-blind study of food extract injection therapy: A preliminary report. Ann Allergy 38:185–191, 1977
66. McEwen LM: Enzyme potentiated hyposensitization. V. Five case reports of patients with acute food allergy. Ann Allergy 35:98–103, 1975

9
Prognosis

In general, the prognosis of sensitivity to cow's milk is excellent, provided milk is effectively eliminated from the diet. Often, however, additional allergens are involved in producing symptoms, and unless they also are identified and avoided, complete relief of symptoms is unlikely. In a series of 59 milk-sensitive infants studied by Gerrard et al.,[1] 20 percent were also allergic to orange, 20 percent to soybean, 12 percent to egg, 8 percent to wheat, 7 percent to tomato, 7 percent to rice, 5 percent to pork meat, 5 percent to lamb meat, and 5 percent to barley.

The duration of sensitivity to milk varies widely from one patient to another, depending partly on age. Its persistence or disappearance is less predictable in adults and older children than in infants. Several follow-up studies[1-4] on infants and young children with milk allergy have shown that allergy to milk often subsides within a few months, and in many instances it disappears or is greatly reduced in severity by 1 to 2 years of age. With maturity of the gastrointestinal tract, the local production of secretory IgA antibodies and other immune systems is believed to be better established, favoring protection and utilization of ingested foreign proteins rather than sensitivity to them. Maturity of the gastrointestinal tract, however, is not always the critical factor; sensitivity to milk may persist throughout adolescence and adulthood, or it may first appear later in life.

Follow-up studies of children who developed milk allergy during early infancy showed that by the end of the first year of life 17 percent[1] to 65 percent[2] were able to tolerate milk in one form or another. The severity of symptoms did not appear to influence the prognosis.[1] When milk sensitivity persists for prolonged periods, new shock organs may become affected or the patient may "outgrow" one symptom only to develop a different one. One study[5] has demonstrated that the course of milk allergy tends to be mild and short in children who had been initially breast-fed and in those who were recognized and given a milk-free diet early.

The goal is to adhere to a strict milk-free diet accompanied by challenge tests every 6 to 18 months to determine whether the sensitivity has declined to a subclinical level. Complete avoidance of milk during the first 6 to 18 months after the diagnosis of milk allergy is made not only is beneficial in rapidly attaining and maintaining an asymptomatic state, but it may also favorably affect the long-term prognosis. Several authors[6-8] described histologic and immunologic abnormalities in the intestinal mucosa after the ingestion of milk in quantities that did not produce clinical symptoms. That finding is important in considering optimal management of milk-sensitive patients who develop minimal or no symptoms while taking small quantities of milk or milk products, especially when milk-related gastroenteropathy or malabsorption was part of the clinical picture. The persistence of intestinal mucosal lesions probably prolongs the duration of milk-sensitivity and leads to insidious digestive disturbances. It may also favor hypersensitivity responses to other ingested antigens and the development of new allergies. In subjects suspected of having milk-related intestinal disease, intestinal biopsy specimens should be examined before and after a challenge test at some time. If the challenge test result is positive, that patient requires particularly careful follow-up because subtle effects from milk ingestion may persist for years or throughout life.

Even after apparent disappearance of sensitivity to milk, most patients seem to be "allergy-prone." Later recurrences or the development of other sensitivities are frequent, and new manifestations may be similar to, or different from, the previous symptoms. Whenever symptoms attributable to allergy occur in a subject who previously was known to be allergic to cow's milk but now seems to tolerate it well, the physician must realize that milk may again have a subtle or a major role in the patient's new symptoms even though they seem unrelated to the earlier milk-related allergy. Therefore, a trial of reeliminating milk from the diet is always in order because it may significantly contribute to the control of the new allergies.

The corollary to that fact is that an inquiry should be made during the workup of every patient with an allergic disease to determine whether a sensitivity to an ingested food, particularly cow's milk, previously existed. If such sensitivity existed, a new trial elimination diet of appropriate duration (usually 1 month) should be accomplished, followed by challenge-testing to demonstrate the presence or absence of persisting (or recurrent) allergy to that food.

REFERENCES

1. Gerrard JW, MacKenzie JWA, Goluboff N, et al.: Cow's milk allergy: Prevalence and manifestations in an unselected series of newborns. Acta Paediatr Scand Suppl 234:1–21, 1973
2. Clein NW: Cow's milk allergy in infants. Pediatr Clin N Am 4:949–962, 1954
3. Gerrard JW, Heiner DC, Ives EJ, et al.: Milk allergy: Recognition, natural history and management. Clin Pediatr 2:634–641, 1963
4. Gryboski JD: Gastrointestinal milk allergy in infants. Pediatrics 40:354–362, 1967
5. Rein D, Shmerling DH: Der Einfluss vorangegangenen Stillens und der Frühdiagnose auf den Krankheitsverlauf bei Kuhmilchprotein-Intoleranz. Helv Paediatr Acta 34:29–40, 1979
6. Savilahti E: Immunochemical study of the malabsorption syndrome with cow's milk intolerance. Gut 14:491–501, 1973
7. Shiner M, Ballard J, Brook CGD, et al.: Intestinal biopsy in the diagnosis of cow's milk protein intolerance without acute symptoms. Lancet 2:1060–1063, 1975
8. Harris MJ, Petts V, Penny R: Cow's milk allegy as a cause of infantile colic: Immunofluorescent studies on jejunal mucosa. Aust Paediatr J 13:276–281, 1977

10
Prevention

Cow's milk allergy is common, especially early in life. It involves many systems of the body, causes a wide variety of symptoms, and frequently imposes difficulties in diagnosis and management. Hence the wisdom in the saying "an ounce of prevention is worth a pound of cure" applies. Because cow's milk allergy is most troublesome during infancy, preventive measures are best instituted at birth or even during pregnancy. The higher the risk of developing allergy, the more important are prophylactic measures. The infant at highest risk of milk allergy is the one whose parents have had milk allergy. When the mother has ongoing allergy to milk, she usually avoids it during pregnancy, which in itself may minimize the likelihood of intrauterine sensitization of the fetus. If only the father has milk allergy, the mother usually does not restrict her intake of cow's milk during either pregnancy or lactation. These factors are discussed in more detail in this chapter.

Prevention of milk allergy has medical, social, and economic advantages. It can reduce the number of doctor visits, the number of admissions to hospitals, the performance of unnecessary diagnostic procedures, and the taking of inappropriate medications. In one study,[1] the percentage of infants with cow's milk allergy who required three or more visits to physicians for illness during the first year of life was 3 times more than that of infants free of allergies, and admissions to hospitals were twice as frequent as were those of the nonallergic infants. The avoidance of any chronic or recurrent illness, such as allergy, will also probably permit a better opportunity for physical and psychologic development, particularly during the formative years of early childhood.

Many studies have reported a lower incidence of allergy in children who were not fed cow's milk during early infancy than in those who were fed cow's milk from birth.[2-5] In one report,[6] the incidence of eczema in cow's milk-fed infants was 7 times that in exclusively breast-fed infants. Saarinen and coworkers[7] and Gruskay[8] recently reported the results of prospective studies that clearly showed that breast-feeding for 6 months or more, especially in babies with a family history of atopy, substantially lowered the incidence of allergic diseases. A study by Halpern et al.,[9] on the other hand, questioned the importance of avoiding feeding cow's milk to newborn infants as a prophylactic measure against allergy. They reported that during the first 6 years of life, the development of allergy was similar in each of three groups fed breast milk, soybean formula, or cow's milk formula during early infancy. Unfortunately, even their breast-fed infants frequently had supplemental cow's milk formula feedings which clouded the overall evaluation of their results. The study was based on data collected from several different practices, and did not provide data on the incidence of allergy during infancy or on the incidence of cow's milk allergy in the various study groups. A second look at the data suggests a higher incidence of cow's milk allergy in the children fed cow's milk. The proportion having cow's milk allergy was 16 percent in the cow's milk-fed allergic group, 12 percent in all allergic children, and, as might be expected, a much lower percentage in the breast-fed allergic group. Their data, however, add weight to the notion that breast-feeding may not prevent the later development of inhalant allergies in atopic children.

A comprehensive approach for preventing milk allergy should use the following techniques:

1. Promotion of the practice of breast feeding
2. Expansion of human-milk banks
3. The use of hypoallergenic formulas or milk substitutes
4. Restriction of intake of cow's milk in high-risk families

Obviously, an effective preventive program cannot be accomplished by the efforts of physicians alone. A successful program requires enthusiastic cooperation between the medical profession, women's organizations, and the infant-food industry.

A Program for Primary Prevention of Cow's Milk Allergy

Promotion of
  Breast-feeding
  Human milk banks
  Hypoallergenic formulas
  Restricted intake of cow's milk in high-risk families
Cooperation of
  Medical profession
    Medical and nursing schools
    Obstetric service

Pediatric service
Maternal and child health clinics
Health educational programs
Women's organizations
Infant-food industry

Modified with permission from Bahna SL: Control of milk allergy: A challenge for physicians, mothers and industry. Ann Allergy 41:1–12, 1978

BREAST-FEEDING

Human milk has proved itself for ages to be the natural and ideal food for the newborn infant. The almost universal decline in the rate and duration of breast-feeding during the twentieth century has been attributed to the wide promotion of formula-feeding, the increased number of working women, and the change in social life-style. Added to these factors, is the diversity of opinion prevailing among the medical profession concerning the value of breast-feeding. Fortunately, the recent upswing in interest in the benefits of breast-feeding has stimulated both the medical profession and the public to consider the advantages of breast-feeding over bottle-feeding.

Interestingly, a rising trend toward breast-feeding has been noted in several industrialized countries, with much of the impetus coming from the better educated women.[10,11] In the United States, the proportion of mothers initiating breast-feeding was around 25 percent in the early 1970s and around 50 percent in 1978.[12,13] More mothers are also continuing to breast-feed for longer periods. In the United States, one study[13] disclosed that the proportion of infants who were breast-fed for 5–6 months or more was 5.5 percent in 1971, 14.7 percent in 1975, and 20.5 percent in 1978. In Sweden, the prevalence of breast-feeding in 1972 was 31 percent at 2 months of age and 6 percent at 6 months of age, and by 1975 the figures had increased to 46 and 14 percent, respectively.[11] In the northern Sydney (Australia) suburbs, in 1972, the rate of breast-feeding on leaving the hospital was 72 percent and at 6 months of age was 12 percent; by 1977 the figures had increased to 86 and 48 percent, respectively.[14]

Advantages of Breast-Feeding

The superiority of breast-feeding has become generally realized, largely because of the lower morbidity and mortality in breast-fed infants than in bottle-fed infants. Such a difference seems to exist in all societies, being more remarkable in less avantaged communities.[15-22] In a recent study, the protective effect of breast-feeding was especially noticeable during the early months of life, increased with the duration of breast-feeding, and operated independently of the socio-educational status, family size, day-care exposure, or birth weight.[23] As the advantages of breast-feeding have become better recognized, pediatric societies have taken a much stronger stand for it than before.[12, 24, 25]

The practice of breast-feeding is advantageous to both the infant and the mother.[12, 26, 32] The advantages of breast-feeding to the infant may be classified into three main groups—nutritional, psychologic, and immunologic.

NUTRITIONAL ADVANTAGES

Nutritional constituents of human milk, cow's milk, and common proprietary formulas are presented in Appendix B, Tables 1 to 4. The nutritional composition of cow's milk in most formulas has been modified to approach that of human milk, and has also been supplemented with vitamins and minerals, a point that is overstressed by manufacturers in promoting formula-feeding. Processed formula is superior to unmodified cow's milk, but human milk still has impressive nutritional advantages over cow's milk formulas.

Nutritional and Socioeconomic Advantages of Breast-feeding

1. Less protein, hence lower nitrogen excretion load
2. Less casein, which is not easily digested
3. Less minerals, hence lower renal solute load
4. Less saturated fatty acids, which are not easily metabolized
5. Ca:P is about 2:1, leading to better Ca absorption
6. More bioavailability of iron
7. Not exposed to errors of preparation
8. No additives or adulteration
9. No preparation, available at any time, fresh, and at body temperature
10. Infant controls quantity, hence less likelihood of overfeeding
11. No cost

Modified with permission from Bahna SL: Control of milk allergy: A challenge for physicians, mothers and industry. Ann allergy 41:1-12, 1978

The digestibility and absorbability of human milk are probably superior, particularly in young infants. The ratio of casein to whey protein is about 2:3 in human milk, compared with 4:1 in cow's milk. Casein curds are somewhat more resistant to digestion in the stomach than are other proteins. The lower content of saturated fatty acids in human milk may also contribute to its easier digestibility.[33-35]

A lower content of methionine and tyrosine and a relatively high content of cystine make human milk more suited for infants and premature infants whose livers are inefficient in converting methionine to cystine or in metabolizing tyrosine.[36] Human milk is also rich in the amino acid taurine, which seems to play a role in neonatal brain growth,[37] as well as in cholesterol and bile acid metabolism.[38]

Minerals in human milk are present in lower concentrations than in cow's milk and thus less solute load is imposed on the immature kidney of the newborn. The low concentration of phosphorous allows a Ca to P ration of about 2:1, which is optimal for intestinal calcium absorption and prevention of neonatal tetany. In cow's milk, calcium and phosphorus are present in almost equal concentrations.

Although the iron concentration in human milk is similar to that in cow's milk, some studies have suggested that iron in human milk has a higher bioavailability.[39-42] Full-term infants who are totally breast-fed may not need iron supplement before 6 months of age.[43]

Human milk contains about 30 mg of cholesterol per 100 ml, compared with 15 to 30 mg/dl in whole cow's milk, and with only 1 to 3 mg/dl in commercial formulas.[44] Breast-fed infants have higher serum concentration of cholesterol than do bottle-fed infants.[43] Because cholesterol is a component of myelin and is a precurser of steroid hormones and of bile acids, the higher cholesterol intake in human milk might possibly be beneficial; strong evidence, however, is lacking.[46]

Thyroid hormones have been detected in human milk but not in cow's milk.[47] Thyroxine and triiodothyronine may be present in concentrations sufficient to alleviate symptoms of hypothyroidism in some breast-fed athyrotic infants,[48] but their presence in breast milk cannot be relied on to prevent the detrimental sequelae of the disease.

In breast-feeding, the intake is primarily under the infant's control, which suits the baby's varying appetite and lessens the problems of overfeeding that may occur with bottle-feeding. In human milk, about 50 percent of the calories are derived from fat, 40 percent from carbohydrate, and 7 percent from protein (the corresponding figures for cow's milk are 50, 30, and 20 percent). The composition of human milk, particularly the lipid content, has shown regular variations during suckling as well as diurnally,[49] which may have a physiological significance to the baby.

Lactating mothers have less tendency to introduce solid foods into the infants's diet at an early time. Not introducing solid food too early helps to avoid gastrointestinal upsets and the development of food allergies. In one study, twice as many formula-fed infants as breast-fed infants were receiving solid foods by 2 months of age.[50]

PSYCHOLOGIC ADVANTAGES

Breast-feeding, when practiced by an interested mother, leads to early, prolonged, and close physical contact between the mother and the infant, which is advantageous to both.[51-55]

Psychologic Advantages of Breast-feeding

Infant
 Is exposed to more intimate sensory stimulation in various modalities
 Develops sense of trust as he is picked up and put at the breast
 Initiates an intimate emotional interaction with the mother
Mother
 Develops self-confidence in mothering
 Fulfills pleasurable instinct
 Promotes emotional stability
 Leads to more affectionate relationship with infant

Modified with permission from Bahna SL: Control of milk allergy: A challenge for physicians, mothers and industry. Ann Allergy 41:1–12, 1978

The dynamics in breast-feeding are unique and cannot be matched by formula-feeding, even more so when the bottle is offered to the baby by persons other than the mother. The process of being picked up, skin-to-skin contact, face-to-face communication, emotional interaction, verbal stimulation, and hearing the mother's heartbeats all provide the infant with optimal sensory stimulation in various modalities including tactile, olfactory, gustatory, visual, and auditory. In endorsing breast-feeding, however, the physcian should be careful not to induce any guilty feelings in mothers who for reasons beyond their control cannot initiate or cannot maintain nursing.

IMMUNOLOGIC ADVANTAGES

Allergy to human milk has never been documented in humans. It was suspected in a few infants more than 3 decades ago[56] but proof was lacking. Interestingly, human milk is devoid of beta-lactoglobulin, the major whey protein and probably the most allergenic component in cow's milk. As far as is known, human milk constituents do not act as foreign antigens to the infant's body. This possible species-specificity has been demonstrated in an experimental model in which it was possible to induce anophylaxis in guinea pigs by bovine or human milks, but not by guinea pig milk.[57] When 10 breast-fed infants with eczema were skin-tested, most had positive reactions to foods that were ingested by the mother, and none reacted to human milk proteins per se;[54] this point is discussed in more detail later in this chapter.

The role played by breast milk in protection against infections is of utmost importance. As early as 1922, Smith and Little[59] reported that about 75 percent of newborn calves deprived of colostrum died of *Escherichia coli* infection, and that the infection could have been prevented by as little as a single ingestion of colostrum. For years gastroenteritis, respiratory infections, meningitis, and gram-negative sepsis have been reported as being less frequent in breast-fed than in bottle fed infants.[20, 22, 60-62] It seems that the anti-infective action of factors in human milk is not limited to the gut. In one study, breast-fed infants showed higher concentrations of secretory IgA in their nasal and salivary secretions in the first few days of life than did formula-fed infants.[63]

Breast milk not only has minimal environmental contamination, but it also contains humoral and cellular elements that impart an anti-infective action.

Immunologic Advantages of Breast-feeding

1. There is much less exposure to ingested allergens
2. Breast milk has minimal exposure to contamination
3. Antibodies (SIgA) protect intestinal mucosa
4. Lactoferrin hinders bacterial growth
5. Lysozyme is antibacterial
6. Lactoperoxidase is antibacterial
7. Bifidus factor promotes desirable intestinal flora
8. Complement enhances chemotaxis and opsonization
9. Antistaphylococcal factor is present
10. Interferon and nonspecific antiviral factors are intact
11. Milk cells: Macrophages, monocytes, neutrophils, B lymphocytes, and T lymphocytes are all present and functional.

Modified with permission from Bahna SL: Control of milk allergy: A challenge for physicians, mothers and industry. Ann Allergy 41:1–12, 1978

These properties obviously make breast-feeding especially desirable in developing countries. Of particular note is the fact that the immunologic components of breast milk are scarcely influenced by the nutritional status of the mother.[64] The anti-infective factors exist in greatly reduced quantities in cow's milk and are largely or totally inactivated in proprietary formulas. Certain characteristics of these factors are summarized in Table 10-1.

Antibodies. All classes of immunoglobulins are present in human milk, with the highest concentrations in colostrum (Table 10-2). The lower concentration in later milk may be compensated for largely by the increase in volume ingested. IgA is the dominant immunoglobulin, and its concentration in colostrum is frequently several times that in the serum, whereas in later milk the concentration is more or less similar to the serum level.[65-70] A recent study has suggested the presence in human colostrum of a factor that enhances the synthesis of IgA by B lymphocytes and has no effect on the production of IgG or IgM.[71] IgA in milk is mostly in the secretory form (SIgA) that resists pH changes and proteolytic enzymes, and thus constitutes a major immunologic defense at the mucosal surface. IgG and IgM concentrations in human milk are usually lower than in the serum, but occasionally colostral IgG and IgM concentrations approach those in the serum.[65] Normally, IgD and IgE are present in low concentrations in colostrum and are barely detectable in late milk.[65,71-74]

Table 10-1
Anti-infective Factors in Human Milk

Factor	Shown in Vitro To Be Active Against	Effect of Heat
Antibacterial		
Lactobacillus bifidus growth factor	Enterobacteriaceae, enteric pathogens	Stable to boiling
Secretory IgA	*Escherichia coli*; *E. coli* enterotoxin; *Clostridium tetani*, *Corynebacterium diphtheriae*, *Diplococcus pneumoniae*, *Salmonella*, *Shigella*	Stable at 56°C for 30 min; some loss (0-30%) at 62.5°C for 30 min; destroyed by boiling
C1-C9	Effect not known	Destroyed by heating at 56°C for 30 min
Lactoferrin	*Escherichia coli*; *Candida albicans*	Two-thirds destroyed at 62.5°C for 30 min
Lactoperoxidase	*Streptococcus*: *Pseudomonas*, *Escherichia coli*, *Salmonella typhimurium*	Not known; presumably destroyed by boiling
Lysozyme	*Escherichia coli*; *Salmonella*, *Mycobacterium lysodeikticus*	Stable at 62.5°C for 30 min; activity reduced 97% by boiling for 15 min
Lipid (unsaturated fatty acid)	*Staphylococcus aureus*	Stable to boiling
Milk cells	By phagocytosis: *Escherichia coli*, *Candida Albicans* By sensitized lymphocytes: *Escherichia coli*	Destroyed by 62.5°C for 30 min
Antiviral		
Secretory IgA	Polio types 1, 2, 3, Coxsackie types A9, B3, B5; Echo types 6, 9; Semliki Forest virus, Ross River virus, rotavirus	Stable at 56°C for 30 min; some loss (0-30%) at 62.5°C for 30 min; destroyed by boiling
Lipid (unsaturated fatty acids and monoglycerides)	Herpes simplex Semliki Forest virus, influenza, dengue, Ross River virus, Murine leukemia virus, Japanese B encephalitis virus	Stable to boiling for 30 min
Nonimmunoglobulin macromolecules	Herpes simplex: vesicular stomatitis virus	Destroyed at 60°C; stable at 56°C for 30 min; destroyed by boiling for 30 min.
	Rotavirus	Unknown
Milk cells	Induced interferon active against Sendai virus; Sensitized lymphocytes? Phagocytosis?	Destroyed at 62.5°C for 30 min

From Welsh JK, May JT: Anti-infective properties of breast milk. J Pediatr 94:1-9, 1979. Reproduced with permission.

Table 10-2
Immunoglobulin, Lysozyme, and Lactoferrin in Colostrum and in Mature Human Milk

Group	Hemoglobin (gm/100 ml)	Serum albumin (gm/100 ml)	IgA (mg/100ml)	IgG (mg/100ml)	IgM (mg/100ml)	Lysozyme (mg/100 ml)	Lactoferrin (mg/100 ml)
Colostrum (1–5 days)							
Well-nourished women	11.5±0.37	2.49±0.065	335.9±37.39 (17)	5.9±1.58 (17)	17.1±4.29 (17)	14.2±2.11 (15)	420±49.0 (28)
Undernourished women	11.3±0.60	2.10±0.081	374.3±42.13 (10)	5.3±2.30 (10)	15.3±2.50 (10)	16.4±2.39 (21)	520±69.0 (19)
Mature milk (1–6 months)							
Well-nourished women	12.8±0.43	3.39±0.120	119.6±7.85 (12)	2.9±0.92 (12)	2.9±0.92 (12)	24.8±3.41 (10)	250±65.0 (17)
Undernourished women	12.6±0.56	3.47±0.130	118.1±16.2 (10)	5.8±3.41 (10)	5.8±3.41 (10)	23.3±3.53 (23)	270±92.0 (13)

Figures in parenthesis indicate number of samples analyzed

From Reddy V, Bhaskaram C, Raghuramulu N, Jagadeeson V: Antimicrobial factors in human milk. Acta Paediatr Scand 66:229-232, 1977. Reproduced with permission.

Human milk contains a wide variety of antibodies, depending on the mother's immunity resulting from immunizations or natural infections. The correlation, however, between antibody titers in milk and in the serum is rather weak. Such antibodies may be against bacteria, bacterial toxins, viruses, and parasites.[66,75-91] In addition to antibodies against infective agents, human milk contains SIgA antibodies directed to food proteins ingested by the mother.[83,87,92-95] These SIgA antibodies may play a significant role in protecting the intestinal mocosa of young infants from penetration by potential food allergens. Hanson et al.[96] noted that breast-fed infants suffering from colic when their mothers drank cow's milk usually had mothers whose breast milk contained no IgA antibodies to cow's milk proteins.

Lactoferrin. The iron-binding whey protein, lactoferrin, was found to have an inhibitory effect on *E. coli* growth, particularly in the presence of antibody,[88,97] also on *Streptoccocus mutans* and *Vibrio cholerae*,[98] as well as on *C. albicans*.[99] The action of lactoferrin is probably through depriving the microorganisms of the ionized iron in the medium.[100]

The concentration of lactoferrin in human milk ranges between 150 and 700 mg/dl, with higher concentration in colostrum than in mature milk.[64,101,102] In cow's milk, lactoferrin is present in small quantities (less than 0.2 mg/dl), and its activity is lost in proprietary formulas. Although saturation of lactoferrin in vitro with iron abolishes its antimicrobial action,[88] iron supplementation to lactating women does not alter the bactericidal activity of breast milk lactoferrin or its degree of saturation.[64] It would be valuable to know whether iron supplementation of breast-fed infants alters the intestinal flora or influences the action of lactoferrin in vivo.

Lysozyme. Lysozyme, or muramidase, is an enzyme that cleaves the cell wall of microorganisms, especialiy of *E. coli* and gram-positive bacteria, and it is present in human milk in a more stable form and in a remarkably higher concentration than in cow's milk.[68,76,102,103]

Lactoperoxidase. The lactoperoxidase system includes the enzyme lactoperoxidase, thiocyanate, and peroxide, and it has been shown to be active against a variety of bacteria such as streptococci, pseudomonas, *E. coli,* and *S. typhimurium.*[104,105] The lactoperoxidase activity in human milk, however, is much less than it is in cow's milk or in the infant's saliva.[104]

Bifidus factor. In contrast to cow's milk, human milk is rich in bifidus factor, which promotes the proliferation of a desirable intestinal flora through facilitating the growth of *L. bifidus* rather than other potentially pathogenic organisms.[80,106] The action of bifidus factor is enhanced by the lactose content, low protein content, low bulk, and low buffering capacity of human milk.[97,107]

Complement. Probably all complement components are present in human milk, although some appear in concentrations higher than others. The C3 and C4 components of complement are present in colostrum in concentrations similar to those in serum, but the levels are much lower in mature milk.[66,68,108] The complement system has a major role in the lysis of bacteria that have been exposed to specific antibody. C3a, a cleavage product of C3, has opsonic, anaphylatoxic, and chemotactic properties. C4 is active in immune adherence. The neutrophil chemotactic activity in colostrum was abolished by heating at 56°C for 60 minutes, but not by lowering the pH to an acidity level similar to that in the stomach of infants.[109] The extent to which complement components in human milk exhibit functional activities in the nursing infant is yet to be defined.

Antistaphylococcal factor. Human milk, but not cow's milk, has been found to increase the resistance of mice to infection with *S. aureus*.[110] The responsible factor is heat-stable and seems to reside in the free fatty acid fraction of milk.

Nonspecific antiviral factors. In addition to specific antiviral antibodies, human milk contains factor(s) with nonspecific antiviral action,[111-113] possibly interferon.[114] These factors are heat-stable and are found largely in the cream rather than in the milk proteins.

Leukocytes. Viable leukocytes exist in human milk in large numbers ranging from 1500 to 3200 cells/cu mm, with greater numbers in colostrum than in mature milk.[76,113,115-117] Most of the cells are macrophages (60 to 90 percent), and the rest are neutrophils and lymphocytes. In colostrum, the lymphocytes are predominantly T cells, whereas in late milk B cells predominate.[118,119]

The macrophages and neutrophils in milk are active in phagocytosis and killing of microorganisms, as well as in producing C3, C4, lysozyme, and lactoferrin.[76,106] Milk lymphocytes are capable of producing IgA[63,76,120] and interferon.[113,121]

Passive transfer of delayed hypersensitivity through breast-feeding has been suggested.[122] A positive tuberculin reaction was observed in 5 out of 9 children who were nursed by tuberculin-positive mothers. Repeated attempts at isolating organisms from the milk of these mothers have failed to demonstrate tubercle bacilli. The mechanism of transfer of delayed hypersensitivity to these infants is unknown. A placental transfer seemed unlikely because the tuberculin reaction was negative in a group of non-breast-fed children of tuberculin-positive mothers. Passage of transfer factor into the milk, or its generation in the gastrointestinal tract of nursing infants, is a possibility.

Mitogenic factor. A mitogenic factor that stimulates DNA synthesis and cell division in mouse and proliferation of human fibroblasts in vitro has been noted in human milk but not in cow's milk or infant formulas.[123,124] This mitogenic activity was much higher in colostrum than in late milk, and was stable at room temperature at pH1 for 2 hours, but was destroyed by trypsin-chymotrypsin digestion. Interestingly, human colostrum contains a trypsin inhibitor.[125] The possible effect of this mitogenic factor on the growth and development on breast-fed infants is not known at the present time.

MATERNAL ADVANTAGES OF BREAST-FEEDING

The advantages to lactating mothers of breast-feeding are multiple and include the following:

1. The psychologic advantages and early establishment of a close relationship with the infant, as was referred to earlier in the chapter.
2. Elimination of the financial burden and effort needed for formula-feeding.
3. Enhancement of the postpartum involution of the uterus.
4. Delay in ovulation, acting as a natural method of contraception. (This advantage is especially important for women who, for financial, religious, or other reasons, do not use other contraceptive measures.)
5. Possibly a lower incidence of breast cancer.[126]

Potential Problems with Breast-feeding

MATERNAL CONDITIONS

1. *Working mothers* may find breast-feeding inconvenient. Milk may be expressed every few hours and kept refrigerated to be fed to the infant while the mother is at work. Supplementary glucose water or a hypoallergenic formula may be given.
2. *Predelivery medication* may influence both the mother's and the infant's ability to initiate breast-feeding for 1 or 2 days. Restriction of the use of sedatives at delivery is advisable.
3. *Breast problems* may be too painful to permit breast-feeding. If the nipples are inverted or sore, milk may be expressed and given in a bottle until the condition improves. If an abscess is present, milk should be expressed from the affected breast and discarded. Nursing from the other breast can be continued unless the baby has a reaction to the antibiotic excreted in milk. Low-grade chronic mastitis may not interfere with breast-feedings, but may elevate sodium and chloride levels in the milk.[127]
4. *Systemic infection,* if contagious, is a contraindication to breast-feeding. The mother should be isolated from the baby and, if her condition permits, the milk may be expressed, boiled, and fed to the baby. Cytomegalovirus,[128,129] hepatitis B virus,[130,131] and rubella virus,[132] have been detected in the milk of asymptomatic mothers, but acquired infection through this route has not been documented. Nevertheless, infection with herpes simplex virus type I via breast milk has been suggested in one infant.[133]

5. *Mental or debilitating diseases* such as postpartum psychosis or advanced cardiac, pulmonary, or renal diseases usually render the mother incapable of nursing. On the other hand, undernutrition usually does not interfere with an adequate milk production.[134] Maternal undernutrition or malnutrition, even when severe, should rarely be a reason to stop breast-feeding: the mother's nutrition, rather, should be corrected.
6. *Oral contraceptives* that contain estrogen-progestin in large amounts tend to suppress lactation. Newer preparations containing progesterone alone do not interfere with milk secretion.[135]
7. *Resumption of menstruation* should not be a reason for discontinuing breast-feeding. Neither should pregnancy during the first 2 to 3 months. Beyond the first trimester, however, nursing is generally an unacceptable additional stress.
8. *An inadequate supply* of breast milk is rarely encountered in the average healthy, emotionally stable mothers. If the baby shows poor weight gain without an obvious cause, supplementation with a hypoallergenic formula is advisable. If supplementation is neglected, hyponatremic dehydration may develop.[136]
9. *Breast cancer virus,* analogous to the B-type RNA tumor virus in certain strains of mice, has been suspected to be present in human milk.[137] No studies have shown any relationship between the presence of such virus particles in milk and the development of breast cancer. A critical review of this subject has been published.[32]

CONDITIONS IN THE INFANT

1. *Oral anomalies* may interfere with successful breast-feeding. Emptying of the breast and feeding the milk by a special nipple or through a gastric feeding tube may suffice until corrective measures are taken. A congenital tooth that is malformed may be extracted. A cleft palate can be fitted with a prosthesis until surgically repaired.
2. *Premature and low-birth-weight* newborn infants are actually the most in need of breast milk. If they cannot suckle from the breast, the milk may be expressed and fed by a dropper, special nipple, or nasogastric tube. In this way, lactation can be maintained until the baby is able to suck the breast. In the face of rapid growth, particularly in infants with a birth weight less than 2000 gm, the usual quantities of breast milk may not supply the infant with all of its needed protein, calcium, phosphorus, sodium, and iron;[138] therefore supplements should be added. Interestingly, analysis of milk samples collected during the first 4 weeks after term and preterm deliveries, revealed that the concentrations of protein, sodium, chloride, and IgA were higher in milk from mothers of preterm infants.[139,140]
3. *Hyperbilirubinemia* may occur in breast-fed infants a few days after birth and persist for several days and occasionally weeks.[141] It is believed to result from inhibition of glucuronyl transferase activity by an unusual metabo-

lite of progesterone (pregnane -3 alpha, 20 beta diol) in colostrum and early milk. Because lipoprotein lipase is present in increased concentrations in milk from nursing mothers of infants with prolonged jaundice,[142] this enzyme has been postulated to have a role also. If the serum bilirubin reaches high levels, substitution of glucose-water for breast-feeding usually results in a rapid decline in bilirubin within 2 to 4 days, after which breast-feeding can be resumed.

4. *Systemic illness,* including erythroblastosis fetalis, should not be a deterrent to breast-feeding unless the infant is acutely ill and cannot suckle the breast, or there is a contraindication to oral feeding. Because human milk has a low concentration of phenylalanine, a diagnosis of phenylketonuria in breast-fed infants may be delayed until the serum phenylalanine level becomes significantly elevated as other foods are introduced into the diet.[143]

5. *Adverse reactions* in exclusively breast-fed infants may result from intake of substances excreted through the breast (Table 10-3). If the mother avoids such substances, the infant's symptoms usually promptly disappear. This subject is discussed in more detail later in this chapter.

6. *Oral poliovirus vaccine* has been reported to have diminished effectiveness in breast-fed infants,[144] probably because of antibodies in the breast milk.[145,146] Whether this interference can be diminished by avoiding breast-feeding for a few hours or a day preadministration or postadministration of the vaccine is not clear. At the present time, the Committee on Infectious Diseases of the American Academy of Pediatrics recommends the same use of oral poliovirus vaccine for both breast-fed and bottle-fed infants.[147]

Table 10-3
Adverse Reactions in Breast-fed Infants

Mechanism	Examples of Offenders
Immunologic	Food antigens
Irritative	Spices, chemicals
Toxic	Drugs, chemicals
Enzyme deficiency	
glucose-6-phosphate dehydrogenase	Fava beans, oxidant drugs
lactase	Lactose

Allergens and Pollutants in Human Milk

Earlier generations believed that the nursing infant could be influenced by the mothers's diet. Later generations considered this belief mere superstition until it became possible to demonstrate in breast milk substances that were ingested by the mother. As found through the use of modern techniques, human milk may contain many substances that the lactating mother has been exposed to in the form of food, drugs, or environmental pollutants. Fortunately, contamination of human milk by substances on the mother's hands or nipple is usually minimal and can be eliminated by cleanliness.

FOODS

In 1918, Talbot[148] reported the development of eczema in a 3-week-old, totally breast-fed infant after the mother had eaten about a pound of chocolate. The eczema cleared when the mother avoided chocolate and it recurred when she ingested cocoa. In 1920, O'Keefe[58] noted that breast-fed infants with eczema may have positive skin reactions to foods that they have never eaten, and in some infants the eczema disappears after the offending food has been eliminated from the mother's diet. Others later have reported similar observations[149,150]

Probably the first demonstration of excretion of food antigens in breast milk was by Shannon,[151] who noted that guinea pigs sensitized to egg protein developed anaphylactic reactions when injected intrathecally with human milk from a nursing woman who was eating eggs but not when she was avoiding them. Intrauterine sensitization of the infant is also a distinct possibility. We, as well as others,[152-155] have observed that antenatal sensitization appears to be triggered in susceptible fetuses by an offending food that has been ingested, sometimes in excessive amounts, by the mother during pregnancy.

Theoretically, any food ingested by a nursing mother could cause ill effects in a susceptible baby. Such effects depend on several factors including the amount of the substance that enters the breast milk in an antigenic or noxious form and the degree of the infant's reactivity. Foods commonly implicated by mothers are spices, cabbage, onions, garlic, turnips, radishes, fish, tomatoes, citrus fruits, rhubarb, and spinach.[26,156] Cow's milk proteins excreted in human milk are seldom considered by nursing mothers to be offenders until milk has been eliminated and then taken again in the diet.[155,157,158] In a series of 19 infants with colic, the symptom disappeared in 13 after cow's milk was eliminated from the mother's diet, and it recurred in 12 after challenge ingestion of milk by the mother.[159] A convincing demonstration of the mechanism is seldom possible in individual instances. Reactions could be immunologic, irritative, toxic, or secondary to an enzyme deficiency. For example, a mother heterozygous for glucose-6-phosphate dehydrogenase deficiency may have a homozygous-affected offspring who develops hemolysis if the mother eats fava beans.[160,161]

The occurrence of these reactions, however, should seldom be a deterrent to breast-feeding, because appropriate modification of the mother's diet usually relieves the infant's symptoms. Only rarely does an infant who is highly sensitive to several foods in the mother's diet need its nutritional intake switched to bottle-feeding. Elimination-challenge diets for the mothers are the keystone of diagnosis. Skilled advice to lactating mothers of infants at high risk for milk allergy may be of preventive value. Similar prophylaxis may be worthwhile during pregnancy because absorbed antigens may cross the placenta in quantities sufficient to sensitize the fetus.

DRUGS

Most drugs taken by the mother are excreted in some form in her milk. Basic drugs (e.g., amphetamine, antihistamines, and erythromycin), or drugs with high lipid solubility (e.g., pentobarbital and secobarbital), tend to concentrate in milk more than do nonionized drugs (e.g., antipyrine, urea, and ethanol).[162,163]

In most instances, drugs taken by the mother are excreted in milk in quantities too small to affect the nursing baby. Ill effects in the infant depend on the dose taken by the mother, the toxicity of the drug, and the individual susceptibility of the infant. Postnatal smoking or alcohol consumption in moderation by the nursing mother has not been documented to cause adverse effects in neonates. On the other hand, heavy smoking or a high intake of alcohol may constitute a risk.[164,165] Caffeine ingested by the mother is excreted in her milk in a concentration of about 50 percent of the serum level and reaches a peak, in both the serum and milk, at 30 to 60 minutes.[166] The maximum quantity of caffeine the lactating mother can take, without causing adverse effects in her infant, is not known. Theophylline appears in milk in a concentration of about 70 percent of the serum level, and its level in the milk peaks about 2 hours after oral intake.[167] Because a nursing infant may occasionally be made irritable by theophylline absorbed via breast milk, an asthmatic mother on full theophylline doses should be advised to nurse her baby before she takes the drug and to avoid nursing 2 to 3 hours after taking the medication.

Drugs known frequently to cause adverse effects in nursing infants are listed below:

Antibacterial: Amantadine, chloramphenicol, nalidixic acid, nitrofurantoin, streptomycin, sulphonamides, tetracyclines
Anticoagulant: Phenindione
Antineoplastic: Cyclophosphamide
Antiparasitic: Metronidazole, quinine
Antithyroid: Iodides, methimazole, propylthiouracil
Cardiovascular: Chlorthalidone, quinidine, reserpine
Diuretic: Hydrochlorothiazide
Gastrointestinal: Purgatives containing cascara, senna, or aloe
Hormones: Corticosteroids, diethylstilbestrol
Neurogenic and Psychogenic: Amphetamine, atropine, bromide, chloral hydrate, chlorpromazine, diazepam, diphenylhydantoin, ergot, heroin, imipramine, lithium, marijuana, methadone, propoxyphene
Miscellaneous: Radioactive agents, lead, mercury, theophylline, tolbutamide

This list is not all-inclusive, but it provides an indication of the scope of the problem. More detailed lists of drugs known to cause or not to cause ill effects in nursing infants have been published in other reviews.[28,32,168-171] Medications for lactating women should be prescribed cautiously and the physician should be alert to the possibility of secondary symptoms in the nursing infant. The health of both the mother and the infant should be considered in deciding which—the medication or the breast-feeding—should be discontinued in the presence of a known risk.

ENVIRONMENTAL POLLUTANTS

Industrial pollutants and pesticides constitute a constant health hazard to human beings, including nursing infants. The presence in human milk of ecologic toxicants, particularly the organochlorine insecticides, is a worldwide phenomenon. Obviously, measures to control such public hazards need to be applied at a community level.

Dichlorodiphenyl-trichloroethane (DDT) concentration in human milk samples from seven cities in the United States ranged from less than 0.02 to 0.83 μg/ml, with a mean of 0.17 μg/ml, whereas the maximum allowable concentration in cow's milk as recommended by the World Health Organization is 0.05 μg/ml.[172] During lactation, women seem to have a negative DDT balance, excreting in their milk about 125 percent of the estimated DDT intake, compared with only 1.5 percent for cattle.[163] Such concentrations do not appear to cause significant ill effects in nursing infants.[173] In socieities that have heavy contamination, however, such as in certain areas of Guatemala,[174] the possibility of later development of adverse effects cannot presently be excluded. The use of DDT has been restricted in certain countries, and a subsequent decrease in its concentration in human milk has been noted in Canada[175] but not in Norway.[176]

Hexachlorobenzene was responsible for an epidemic of toxic symptoms in Turkey in 1956 in nursing infants whose mothers had eaten contaminated wheat.[177] A similar epidemic caused by *methylmercury* occurred in Iraq in 1972.[178]

Dieldrin, hexachlorocyclohexane, and *heptachlorepoxide* have been found in various concentrations in human milk, but less frequently than have certain other insecticides.[176,179]

Polychlorinated biphenyls (PCBs), a worldwide industrial pollutant, has also been detected in human milk. Under usual circumstances the concentration in milk is too small to cause symptoms. The later development of ill effects has not been explored.[180,181] On the other hand, after exposures, such as in the Japanese epidemic of 1968, clinical adverse effects have persisted for months or years.[182]

Polybrominated biphenyls (PBBs) also is an industrial pollutant, and like

PCBs is a potential contaminant in foods that may be marketed for human consumption. An outbreak occurred in farming animals in Michigan in 1973.[183] Although it is excreted in various concentrations in milk, ill effects in nursing infants have not been documented.

Human-milk Banking

Human-milk banking should be a basic component of any community program promoting breast-feeding. Such banks have been available in many countries, mostly initiated by the efforts of interested local medical centers. In most instances, milk is obtained from volunteer donors and distributed on a limited scale. Priorities of distribution have usually been given to preterm or sick neonates, or to newborn infants whose mothers have problems that temporarily interfere with breast-feeding. Distribution on a larger scale is expected to follow an increase in the number of lactating women and donors.

The requirements for a successful human-milk banking system are enthusiastic physicians, nurses, and women's organizations that promote breast-feeding and recruitment of milk donors, and the technology of an interested infant-food industry that provides proper collection, processing, storage, and distribution. Recruitment of volunteer donors would be best initiated in maternity clinics and wards through written and verbal messages tactfully delivered by physicians or nurses. Poster campaigns, articles in newspapers and women's magazines, and spot messages on radio and television can be used to sustain momentum and engender public enthusiasm.

The ideal method of processing human milk has not yet been developed.[184,185] Standards are needed to guarantee bacterial safety and minimal alteration in milk quality, particularly in its immunologic integrity.

Milk should be expressed from the breast with utmost cleanliness into sterile containers, and immediately refrigerated if its ransfer to the bank will be within 24 hours; otherwise it should be put in a freezer. Expression of milk at the bank itself would be ideal, but this is often not practical. Instructions for hygienic measures for collecting milk should be given both verbally and in writing. The first 5 to 10 ml of expressed milk should not be banked because its omission would reduce the bacterial count by 10- to 100-fold.[186] Initial and periodic home visits by a nurse will be both supportive and valuable in discovering contraindications to milk collection from certain donors. Screening of all new donors for hepatitis B antigen is desirable,[186] even though transmission of this disease through breast-feeding has not been documented. Collection of milk should be stopped if the donor or her baby is ill, or if she is taking medication likely to cause ill effects in infants fed that milk (see list on p. 156).

Methods used for processing human milk include heat treatment, lyophilization, freezing, and gamma irradiation. Heating above 70°C is detrimental to the immunologic properties of human milk.[187-189] Boiling also increases the osmolality, particularly of colostrum, imposing a high solute load on newborn infants.[186] Holder pasteurization (62.5°C for 30 min) and gamma irradiation are equally effective in killing bacteria, but gamma irradiation denatures IgA and lactoferrin.[188]

The effects of holder pasteuirzation, lyophilization, and freezing on the immunologic components of human milk are compared in Table 10-4. IgA is slightly affected by any of the three methods. The loss in IgG is moderate during pasteurization or lyophilization, and is minimal by freezing. One study, based on a small number of samples, reported a moderate loss in IgM by pasteurization and a great loss by lyophilization or freezing.[190] Pasteurization inactivates C3 and most of lactoferrin, whereas lysozyme is fairly stable to all three methods. Lymphocytes in milk are highly sensitive to any of the three methods of treatment.

Freezing would appear to be the ideal method when milk is collected under strict aseptic conditions and stored immediately in a freezer until gently thawed just before feeding. Breast milk collected in centers by trained personnel and under specified conditions has a better bacteriologic quality than milk expressed by donors at home.[192] Pasteurization, though not ideal, seems to be the most acceptable method in most instances at the present time. Unless it is for immediate use, pasteurized milk should be stored frozen until needed. Raw human milk that contains commensal organisms only, is probably safe for feeding healthy newborns.[193] Its use in feeding preterm infants, however, is still debatable; it has been favored by some investigators[186] and opposed by others.[194]

The ability of lymphocytes to survive in the infant's stomach[117] raises an important question about the desirability of feeding viable lymphocytes in milk from a woman other than the mother.[195] For human milk to retain viable lymphocytes, it should be collected in plastic containers and kept at room temperature and at a pH between 3.0 and 7.0

OTHER MILK SUBSTITUTES

If human milk cannot be provided to a newborn infant, a hypoallergenic formula is preferred over cow's milk formula. A hypoallergenic formula is especially recommended for the potentially allergic infant, i.e., the infant with at least one allergic parent or sibling, and is strongly recommended if anyone in the immediate family has had prior milk allergy. Preparations that may be used for this purpose include the following:

Soybean formula
Casein hydrolysates
Evaporated cow's milk
Elemental diet
Meat-base formula

Table 10-4
Effect of Holder Pasteurization, Lyophilization, and Freezing on the Immunologic Components of Human Milk

Component	Pasteurization % loss	Pasteurization References	Lyophilization % loss	Lyophilization References	Freezing % loss	Freezing References
IgA	0 to 23	187–190	2 to 21	189,190	3 to 14	189,190
IgG	34 to 61	189 190	21 to 68	189,190	0	189
IgM	Moderate*	190	Great*	190	Great*	190
C3	100	91	6	189	7	189
Lactoferrin	44 to 62	187,189,191	0	189	0	189
Lysozyme	0 to 24	187,189,191	6	189	10	189
Anti-*E. coli*	Slight to moderate	190,191	Moderate	190	Slight	190
α1 Antitrypsin	34	191	7	189	17	189
Lymphocytes	100	190	100	190	100	190

*The sample size was small and actual figures were not available.

These preparations have been discussed earlier, in Chapter 8.

Soybean formula has been the most commonly used preparation for prophylaxis against cow's milk allergy. In 1952, Glaser and Johnstone[196] reported a series of 67 potentially allergic infants who were successfully fed soy formula from birth. The same authors, in a retrospective study,[2,197] noted in a group of potentially allergic children who were fed mostly soybean preparation from birth and were not given cow's milk for varying periods during infancy, that by 6 years of age the incidence of major allergies was about one-fourth that of cow's-milk-fed siblings (15 vs. 65 percent). This observation was supported later by a prospective 10-year follow-up study by Johnstone and Dutton.[3] Of potentially allergic children who were fed soybean formula from birth and were not given bovine products, chicken, egg, or wheat during the first 9 months of life, 18 percent developed respiratory allergies compared with 50 percent of the cow's-milk-fed group. In a study that was not restricted to potentially allergic infants, however, the incidence of allergy during a follow-up period of 12 to 27 months was 10.6 percent in a group fed soybean formula and 13.3 percent in a group given cow's milk.[198]

In a study of circulating antibodies in young infants, soy protein and cow's milk protein were found to have equal antigenicity.[199] That study, however, did not demonstrate equal allergenicity of the two kinds of proteins. Other authors reported no advantage of soybean formula over cow's milk formula in the prophylaxis against allergic diseases in general.[8,200]

INTRODUCTION OF OTHER FOODS

During the first 6 months of life, most infants grow well on human milk and/or a hypoallergenic formula alone. After 6 months of age, other foods may be introduced, beginning with rice, barley, and oat cereals; juices, fruits, and vegetables; and lamb, and beef. Eggs, fish, and cow's milk and its products, are better avoided until 9 to 12 months of age.

New foods should be added one at a time and not more than one new food every week. Single food items rather than combinations should be used. In this way, if an adverse reaction develops, the offending food can be easily identified. Cow's milk, when first introduced, should be in a heat-treated form (evaporated or boiled for 10 min). Unboiled homogenized pasteurized milk is not recommended before the age of 1 year.

ROLE OF THE MEDICAL PROFESSION

The prevention of illness is a major responsiblity of the health profession as well as of conscientious parents. The primary concern of many physicians, however, has been therapy rather than prevention. In working to prevent milk allergy and other ill effects of using cow's milk for infant feeding, the medical profession should address itself to several areas, including the following:

1. *Undergraduate teaching* in both medical and nursing schools should emphasize the importance of breast-feeding. Students should also be taught to participate in the education of the public concerning breast-feeding.
2. *Creating positive attitudes* toward breast-feeding. Physicians and nurses working in obstetrics, newborn nurseries, pediatrics, family practice, and well-baby clinics are in a favorable position to endorse breast-feeding. Caution should be practiced in order to avoid creating guilty feelings in parents who decide not to breast-feed. Women who decide to breast-feed, especially those who have not breast-fed before, should be given information on antenatal breast care and on the practical aspects of breast-feeding.[201, 202] Mothers can also find a great help from reading about breast-feeding.[201, 207] Breast-feeding should be maintained as much as possible of the first 9 to 12 months of life.
3. *Maternity centers* should encourage breast-feeding. In-hospital instruction by enthusiastic personnel has a very favorable influence on increasing the rate of breast-feeding.[208-210] Unfortunately, the policy of some maternity wards discourages or even opposes breast-feeding for the convenience of the nursing staff. It would be appropriate if hospitals would require informed consent of parents, obtained by both the obstetrician and pediatrician, before formula-feeding is ordered for the newborn infant.
4. *Health educational programs,* particularly those directed to adolescent girls and young women, should emphasize the advantages of the natural mode of infant feeding.
5. *Editors of medical journals* should assume responsibility for seeing that advertisements submitted by manufacturers of formulas are well screened.

ROLE OF WOMEN'S ORGANIZATIONS

Every mother wishes her baby to have the best possible food. The importance of participation by women's organizations in promoting breast-feeding cannot be overemphasized. One large organization that has shown leadership in this respect is La Leche League International*, which began in the United States about a quarter of a century ago and now has worldwide activities helping mothers, nurses, and physicians to promote breast-feeding.[211] Expectant and lactating mothers can obtain valuable help from members of La Leche in their localities. The Human Lactation Center, Ltd.† is another organization with similar interest.

*La Leche League International, 9616 Minneapolis Ave., Franklin Park, Ill., 60131, U.S.A.
†The Human Lactation Center, Ltd., 666 Sturgis Highway, Westport, Conn., 06880, U.S.A.

Activities that can be adopted by women's organizations to promote breast-feeding include the following:

1. *Hold group meetings* to discuss various aspects of breast-feeding. Such discussions should be moderated by selected persons capable of delivering convincing facts. A special effort should be made to invite pregnant and lactating women so that questions can be answered and fears alleviated.
2. *Have individual counseling* of pregnant women and new mothers by others who have successfully breast-fed. Young women are more likely to be influenced by lactating women of similar age, or by those who are only slightly older, than by older women.
3. *Distribute information* through pamphlets, booklets, articles in women's magazines, radio, television, and newspapers.
4. *Support hospitals that favor breast-feeding.* It is the women's right to deliver in maternity wards that encourage breast-feeding and to boycott those that do not.
5. *Demand modified working conditions* to maintain breast-feeding. Lactating women may be granted 3 to 9 months materntiy leave. Establishment of sufficient numbers of day-care nurseries in business areas of cities will encourage working mothers to nurse their babies during the day.
6. *Support human-milk banking* through the recruitment of donors.

When breast-feeding has been generally accepted in developed countries, the Western woman will not only reap the fruit of good health in her own children but also will become an example to women in developing countries, where the need for breast-feeding is even greater.

ROLE OF INFANT-FOOD INDUSTRY

The food industry has been blamed for manipulating the practice of infant feeding. Formula-manufacturers are especially criticized for their inappropriate promotional activities that reach even the most backward regions of developing countries, resulting in grave consequences.[212-214]

Moreover, the food industry has assumed a leadership role in supplying information on nutrition, both to the public and to health professionals. The profit-making incentive should not be allowed to diminish the food industry's concern for the people's health or a nation's economy. Sales representatives should not be concerned only with selling as much of a product as possible. Methods of advertisement that have been used to influence the medical profession, hospitals, and the public should be carefully scrutinized. The mass media are flooded with advertisements on infant formulas stamped with the famous sign of a smiling plump baby. Maternity wards are given generous donations of cow's milk formulas. On discharge from the hospital, "starter samples" of formulas and persuasive information for bottle-feeding are distributed to parturient women, even to those who want to breast-feed. In rural areas of the Philippines, for example, 41 percent of women who delivered in hospitals were given free samples of formula.[215]

Probably because of recent rising criticism, the infant-food industry has formed the International Council of Infant Food Industries.[216] This council comprises representatives of many formula-producing companies, and aims to become a self-regulating agency of the infant-food industry throughout the world. Because of past performance and the need for outside participation and direction, this council has not been well received by health professionals.[214]

It is time for manufacturers of formulas to reconsider their policies and to show more concern for child health. With that goal in mind, the infant-food industry must consider several issues:

1. *A substantial change in advertising policy* is needed. Equality between formula and human milk feeding must not be claimed. Promotional activities should be supervised by noncommercially committed health professionals and informed members of the public. Codes of ethics have been recently adopted by the infant-food manufacturers.[217]
2. *Inexpensive, nutritionally adequate formulas* should be available for infants who cannot be provided with human milk.
3. *Hypoallergenic formulas* with minimal additives and at low cost are needed for feeding potentially allergic infants and those sensitive to cow's milk.
4. *Nutritional supplements* for infants and for undernourished pregnant or lactating women would be widely welcomed, particularly in developing countries. Accurate and complete labeling of the constituents and mode of preparation of all such formulas would be very valuable, especially for those suffering from any form of allergy.[218]
5. *Human-milk banking* needs the technologic expertise of the food industry especially for developing the optimal method for processing human milk.

The need is urgent for the medical profession and the infant-food industry to unite in assisting mothers to practice better infant-feeding.[219] Governments in both developing and industrialized countries must assume responsibility for issuing and enforcing regulations that more firmly place their children on the road of physical health and emotional well-being.

REFERENCES

1. Gerrard JW, MacKenzie JWA, Goluboff N, et al.: Cow's milk allergy: Prevalence and manifestations in an unselected series of newborns. Acta Paediatr Scand Suppl 234:1–21, 1973
2. Glaser J, Johnstone DE: Prophylaxis of allergic disease in newborn. JAMA 153:620–622, 1953

3. Johnstone DE, Dutton AM: Dietary prophylaxis of allergic diseases in children. N Engl J Med 274:715–719, 1966
4. Soothill JF: Some intrinsic and extrinsic factors predisposing to allergy. Proc R Soc Med 69:439–442, 1976
5. Kaufman HS, Frick OL: The incidence of asthma in bottle and breast fed infants: A prospective study. Ann Allergy 42:128, 1979
6. Grulee CG, Sanford HN: The influence of breast and artificial feeding on infantile eczema. J Pediatr 9:223–225, 1936
7. Saarinen UM, Backman A, Kajosaari M, et al.: Prolonged breast-feeding as prophylaxis for atopic disease. Lancet 2:163–166, 1979
8. Gruskay FL: Prophylaxis of allergic disease. Does milk-free diet help? A prospective study. X International Congress of Allergology, Jerusalem, November 4–11, 1979, p 129
9. Halpern SR, Sellars WA, Johnson RB, et al.: Development of childhood allergy in infants fed breast, soy or cow milk. J Allergy Clin Immunol 51:139–151, 1973
10. Jelliffe DB: World trends in infant feeding. Am J Clin Nutr 29:1227–1237, 1976
11. Hofvander Y, Petros-Barvazian A: WHO collaborative study on breast feeding. Acta Paediatr Scand 67:556–560, 1978
12. American Academy of Pediatrics, Committee on Nutrition: Breast-feeding. Pediatrics 62:591–601, 1978
13. Martinez GA, Nalezienski JP: The recent trend in breast-feeding. Pediatrics 64:686–692, 1979
14. Lawson JS, Mays CA, Oliver TI: The return to breast feeding. Med J Aust 2:229–230, 1978
15. Woodbury RM: The relation between breast and artificial feeding and infant mortality. Am J Hygiene 2:668–687, 1922
16. Grulee CG, Sanford HN, Herron PH: Breast and artificial feeding. JAMA 103:735–739, 1934
17. Stevenson SS: Adequacy of artificial feeding in infancy. J Pediatr 31:616–630, 1947
18. Naish FC: Morbidity and feeding in infancy. Lancet 1:146, 1949
19. Robinson M: Infant morbidity and mortality: Study of 3,266 infants. Lancet 1:788–794, 1951
20. Winberg J, Wessner G: Does breast milk protect against septicemia in the newborn? Lancet 1:1091–1094, 1971
21. Downham MAPS, Scott R, Sims DG, et al.: Breast-feeding protects against respiratory syncytial virus infection. Br Med J 2:274–276, 1976
22. Cunningham AS: Morbidity in breast-fed and artificially-fed infants. J Pediatr 90:726–729, 1977
23. Cunningham AS: Morbidity in breast-fed and artificially fed infants. II. J Pediatr 95:685–689, 1979
24. American Academy of Pediatrics, Committee on Nutrition: Commentary on breast-feeding and infant formulas, including proposed standards for formulas. Pediatrics 57:278-285, 1976
25. Farmer K, Begg NC, Birkbeck JA, et al.: Breastfeeding: A Statement of the Infant Nutrition Subcommittee of the Paediatric Society of New Zealand. NZ Med J 86:144–147, 1977
26. Harfouche JK: The importance of breast-feeding. J Trop Pediatr 16:133–175, 1970
27. Jelliffe DB: Unique properties of human milk: Remarks on some recent developments. J Reprod Med 14:133–137, 1975
28. Oseid BJ: Breast-feeding and infant health. Clin Obstet Gynecol 18:149–173, 1975
29. Jelliffe DB, Jelliffe EFP: "Breast is best": Modern meanings. N Engl J Med 297:912–915, 1977
30. Nestlé Editorial Committee: Breast-Feeding. Annales Nestlé, vol 39, Vevey, Switzerland, Nestlé, 1977
31. Taylor B: Breast versus bottle feeding. NZ Med J 85:235–238, 1977
32. Wing JP: Human versus cow's milk in infant nutrition and health. Curr Probl Pediatr 8:1–50, 1977

33. Fomon SJ, Ziegler EE, Thomas LN, et al.: Excretion of fat by normal full-term infants fed various milks and formulas. Am J Clin Nutr 23:1299–1313, 1970
34. Belavady B: Lipid and trace element composition of human milk. Acta Paediatr Scand 67:566–571, 1978
35. Jensen RG, Hagerty MM, McMahon KE: Lipids of human milk and infant formulas: A review. Am J Clin Nutr 31:990–1016, 1978
36. Raiha NCR: Biochemical basis for nutritional management of preterm infants. Pediatrics 53:147–156, 1974
37. Rassin DK, Sturman JA, Gaull GE: Taurine in milk: Species variation. Pediatr Res 11:449, 1977
38. Rassin DK, Jarvenpaa A-L, Raiha NCR, et al.: Breast-feeding versus formula feeding in full-term infants: Effects on taurine and cholesterol. Pediatr Res 13:406, 1979
39. McMillan JA, Landaw SA, Oski FA: Iron sufficiency in breast-fed infants and the availability of iron from human milk. Pediatrics 58:686–691, 1976
40. Saarinen UM, Siimes MA, Dalhman PR: Iron absorption in infants: High bioavailability of breast milk iron as indicated by the extrinsic tag method of iron absorption and by the concentration of serum ferritin. J Pediatr 91:36–39, 1977
41. Woodruff CW, Latham C, McDavid S: Iron nutrition in the breast-fed infant. J Pediatr 90:36–39, 1977
42. Saarinen UM, Siimes MA: Iron absorption from breast milk, cow's milk, and iron-supplemented formula: An opportunistic use of changes in total body iron determined by hemoglobin, ferritin, and body weight in 132 infants. Pediatr Res 13:143–147, 1979
43. Saarinen UM: Need for iron supplementation in infants on prolonged breast feeding. J Pediatr 93:177–180, 1978
44. Glueck CJ: A pediatric approach in high risk infants to the primary prevention of atherosclerosis, in Filer LJ Jr, Brasel JA, Glueck CJ, et al. (eds): Infant Nutrition, part 2. Bloomfield, N.J., Health Learning Systems Inc., 1977, pp 27–34
45. Darmady JM, Fosbrooke AS, Lloyd JK: Prospective study of serum cholesterol levels during first year of life. Br Med J 2:685–688, 1972
46. Fomon SJ: Infant Nutrition (ed 3). Philadelphia, Saunders, 1974, p 174
47. Varma SK, Collins M, Row A, et al.: Thyroxine, tri-iodothyronine, and reverse tri-iodothyronine concentration in human milk. J Pediatr 93:803–806, 1978
48. Bode HH, Vanjonack WJ, Crawford JD: Mitigation of cretinism by breast feeding. Pediatrics 62:13–16, 1978
49. Hall B: Uniformity of human milk. Am J Clin Nutr 32:304–312, 1979
50. Sleigh G, Ounsted M: Present-day practice in infant feeding. Lancet 1:753, 1975
51. Stone S, Bakwin H: Psychologic aspects of pediatrics: Breast-feeding. J Pediatr 33:660–667, 1948
52. Newton N: Psychologic differences between breast and bottle feeding. Am J Clin Nutr 24:993–1004, 1971
53. Klaus MH, Jerauld R, Kreger NC, McAlpine W, et al.: Maternal attachment: Importance of the first post-partum days. N Engl J Med 286:460–463, 1972
54. Salk L: The role of the heartbeat in the relation between mother and infant. Sci Am 228:24–29, 1973
55. Kennell J, Jerauld R, Wolfe H, et al.: Maternal behavior one year after early and extended post-partum contact. Dev Med Child Neurol 16:172–179, 1974
56. Wergeland H: Three fatal cases of probable familial allergy to human milk. Acta Paediatr Scand 35:321–334, 1948
57. Campbell SG, Vier EJ: The immunogenicity of milk from various species for the guinea-pig. Clin Exp Immunol 33:514–518, 1978
58. O'Keefe ES: The relation of food to infantile eczema. Boston Med Surg J 183:569–573, 1920

59. Smith T, Little RB: The significance of colostrum to the new-born calf. J Exp Med 36: 181–198, 1922
60. Mellander O, Vahlquist B, Mellbin T: Breast feeding and artificial feeding: A clinical, serological and biochemical study on 402 infants, with a survey of the literature. The Norrbotten study. Acta Paediatr Scand 48 (Suppl 116): 1–99, 1959
61. Ironside AG, Tuxford AF, Heyworth B: A survey of infantile gastroenteritis. Br Med J 3:20–24, 1970
62. Larsen SA Jr., Homer DR: Relation of breast versus bottle feeding in hospitalization for gastroenteritis in a middle class U.S. population. J Pediatr 92:417–418, 1978
63. Roberts SA, Freed DLJ: Neonatal IgA secretion enhanced by breast-feeding. Lancet 2:1131, 1977
64. Reddy V, Bhaskaram C, Raghuramulu N., et al.: Antimicrobial factors in human milk. Acta Paediatr Scand 66:229–232, 1977
65. Heiner DC: Biological, immunological and physiochemical properties of γD immunoglobulin (IgD). A thesis in partial fulfillment of the degree of Doctor of Philosophy. McGill University, Montreal, 1969
66. Mata LJ, Wyatt RG: Host resistance to infection. Am J Clin Nutr 24:976–986, 1971
67. Hanebery B: Human milk immunoglobulins and agglutinins to rabbit erythrocytes. Int Arch Allergy Appl Immunol 47:716–729, 1974
68. McClelland DBL, McGrath J, Samson RR: Antimicrobial factors in human milk: Studies of concentration and transfer to the infant during the early stages of lactation. Acta Paediatr Scand Suppl 271:3–20, 1978
69. Ogra SS, Ogra PL: Immunologic aspects of human colostrum and milk. I. Distribution characteristics and concentrations of immunoglobulins at different times after the onset of lactation. J Pediatr 92: 546–549, 1978
70. Önes SÜ: Immunoglobulins of human colostrum and milk. J Pediatr 94:497–498, 1979
71. Pittard WB III, Bill K: Immunoregulation by breast milk cells. Cellular Immunol 42:437–441, 1979
72. Underdown BJ, Knight A, Papsin FR: The relative paucity of IgE in human milk. J Immunol 116:1435–1438, 1976
73. Turner MW, McClelland DBL, Medlen AR, et al.: IgE in human urine and milk. Scand J Immunol 6:343–348, 1977
74. Bahna SL, Keller MA, Heiner DC: IgE and IgD in human milk and plasma. In manuscript
75. Hanson LÅ, Winberg J: Breast milk and defense against infection in the newborn. Arch Dis Child 47:845–848, 1972
76. Goldman AS, Smith CW: Host resistance factors in human milk. J Pediatr 82:1082–1090, 1973
77. Ste-Marie MT, Lee EM, Brown WR: Radioimmunologic measurements of naturally occurring antibodies. III. Antibodies reactive with *Escherichia coli* or *Bacteroides fragilis* in breast fluids and sera of mothers and newborn infants. Pediatr Res 8:815–819, 1974
78. Carlsson B, Gothefors L, Ahlstedt S, et al.: Studies of *Escherichia coli* O antigen specific antibodies in human milk, maternal serum and cord blood. Acta Paediatr Scand 65:216–224, 1976
79. Carlsson B, Ahlstedt S, Hanson LÅ, et al.: *Escherichia coli* O antibody content in milk from healthy Swedish mothers and mothers from a very low socio-economic group of a developing country. Acta Paediatr Scand 65:417–423, 1976
80. Bullen JJ: Iron-binding proteins and other factors in milk responsible for resistance to *Escherichia coli*. Ciba Found Symp 42:149–169, 1976
81. Holmgren J, Hanson LÅ, Carlsson B, et al.: Neutralizing antibodies against *Escherichia coli* and *Vibrio cholerae* enterotoxins in human milk from a developing country. Scand J Immunol 5:867–871, 1976

82. Stoliar OA, Pelley RP, Kaniecki-Green E, et al.: Secretory IgA against enterotoxins in breast-milk. Lancet 1:1258–1261, 1976
83. Ahlstedt S, Carlsson B, Fällström SP, et al.: Antibodies in human serum and milk induced by enterobacteria and food proteins. Ciba Found Symp 46:115–134, 1977
84. Santoro F, Borojevic R, Bout D, et al.: Mother-child relationship in human schistosomiasis mansoni. I. Parasitic antigens and antibodies in milk. Am J Trop Med Hyg 26:1164–1168, 1977
85. Schoub BD, Prozesky OW, Lecatsas G, et al.: The role of breast-feeding in the prevention of rotavirus infection. J Med Microbiol 11:25–31, 1977
86. Thouless ME, Bryden AS, Flewett TH: Rotavirus neutralisation by human milk. Br Med J 2:1390, 1977
87. Hanson LÅ, Ahlstedt S, Carlsson B, et al.: New knowledge in human milk immunoglobulin. Acta Paediatr Scand 67:577–582, 1978
88. Rogers HJ, Synge C: Bacteriostatic effect of human milk on *Escherichia coli:* The role of IgA. Immunology 34:19–28, 1978
89. Welsh JK, Skurrie IJ, May JT: Use of semliki forest virus to identify lipid-mediated antiviral activity and anti-alphavirus immunoglobulin A in human milk. Infect Immun 19:395–401, 1978
90. Cukor G, Blacklow NR, Capozza FE, et al.: Persistence of antibodies to rotavirus in human milk. J Clin Microbiol 9:93–96, 1979
91. Welsh JK, May JT: Anti-infective properties of breast milk. J Pediatr 94:1–9, 1979
92. McClelland DBL, McDonald TT: Antibodies to dietary proteins in human colostrum. Lancet 2:1251–1252, 1976
93. Hanson DG, Vaz NM, Maia LCS, et al.: Tolerance to proteins induced by feeding. Ann Allergy 38:386, 1977
94. Soothill JF: Immunodeficiency, allergy and infant feeding, in Hambraeus L, Hanson LÅ, McFarlane HM (eds): Food and Immunology. Swedish Nutrition Foundation Symposia Series XIII, Stockholm, Almquist & Wiksell International, 1977, p 148
95. Walker WA: Development of intestinal host defense mechanisms and the passive protective role of human milk. Mead Johnson Symp Perinat Dev Med 11:39–48, 1977
96. Hanson LÅ, Ahlstedt S, Carlsson B, et al.: Secretory IgA antibodies against cow's milk proteins in human milk and their possible effect in mixed feeding. Int Arch Allergy Appl Immunol 54:457–462, 1977
97. Bullen CL, Willis AT: Resistance of the breast-fed infant to gastroenteritis. Br Med J 3:338–343, 1971
98. Arnold RR, Cole MF, McGhee JR: A bactericidal effect for human lactoferrin. Science 197:263–265, 1977
99. Kirkpatrick CH, Green I, Rich RR, et al.: Inhibition of growth of *Candida albicans* by iron-unsaturated lactoferrin: Relation to host defense mechanisms in chronic mucocutaneous candidiasis. J Infect Dis 124:539–544, 1971
100. Oram JD, Reiter B: Inhibition of bacteria by lactoferrin and other iron-chelating agents. Biochim Biophys Acta 170:351–366, 1968
101. Masson PL, Heremans JF: Lactoferrin in milk from different species. Comp Biochem Physiol 39:119–129, 1971
102. Hambraeus L, Lönnerdal B, Forsum E, et al.: Nitrogen and protein components of human milk. Acta Paediatr Scand 67:561–565, 1978
103. Chandan RC, Shahani KM, Holly RG: Lysozyme content of human milk. Nature (Lond) 204:76–77, 1964
104. Gothefors L, Marklund S: Lactoperoxidase activity in human milk and saliva of the newborn infant. Infect Immunol 11:1210–1215, 1975
105. Björk L, Rosen CG, Marshall V, et al.: Antibacterial activity of the lactoperoxidase system in

milk against pseudomonads and other gram-negative bacteria. Appl Environ Microbiol 30:199–204, 1975
106. Mata LJ, Urrutia JJ: Intestinal colonization of breast-fed children in a rural area of low socioeconomic level. Ann NY Acad Sci 176:93–109, 1971
107. Heine W, Zunft HJ, Müller-Beuthow W, et al.: Lactose and protein absorption from breast milk and cow's milk preparations and its influence on the intestinal flora. Acta Paediatr Scand 66:699–703, 1977
108. Jagadeesan V, Reddy V: C3 in human milk. Acta Paediatr Scand 67:237–238, 1978
109. Björksten B, Gothefors L, Sidenvall R: The effects of human colostrum on neutrophil function. Pediatr Res 13:737–741, 1979
110. György P, Dhanamitta S, Steers E: Protective effects of human milk in experimental staphylococcal infection. Science 137:338–340, 1962
111. Falker WA Jr, Diwan AR, Halstead SB: A lipid inhibitor of dengue virus in human milk; with a note on the absence of antidengue secretory antibody. Arch Virol 47:3–10, 1975
112. Matthew THJ, Nair CDG, Lawrence MK, et al.: Antiviral activity in milk of possible clinical importance. Lancet 2:1387–1389, 1976
113. Lawton JWM, Shortridge KF: Protective factors in human breast milk and colostrum. Lancet 1:253, 1977
114. Lawton JM, Shortridge KF, Wong RC, et al.: Interferon synthesis by human colostral leukocytes. Arch Dis Child 54:127–130, 1979
115. Mohr JA, Liu R, Mabry W: Colostral leukocytes. J Surg Oncol 2:163–167, 1970
116. Robinson JE, Harvey BAM, Soothill JF: Phagocytosis and killing of bacteria and yeast by human milk cells after opsonization in aqueous phase of milk. Br Med J 1:1443–1445, 1978
117. Paxson CL Jr, Cress CC: Survival of human milk leukocytes. J Pediatr 94:61–64, 1979
118. Parmely MJ, Beer AE, Billingham RE: In vitro studies on the T-lymphocyte population of human milk. J Exp Med 144:358–370, 1976
119. Ogra SS, Ogra PL: Immunologic aspects of human colostrum and milk. II. Characteristics of lymphocyte reactivity and distribution of E-rosette forming cells at different times after the onset of lactation. J Pediatr 92:550–555, 1978
120. Pittard WB III, Polmar SH, Fanaroff AA: The breastmilk macrophage: A potential vehicle for immunoglobulin transport. J Reticuloendothel Soc 22:597–603, 1977
121. Emodi G, Just M: Interferon production by lymphocytes in human milk. Scand J Immunol 3:157–159, 1974
122. Mohr JA: The possible induction and/or acquisition of cellular hypersensitivity associated with ingestion of colostrum. J Pediatr 82:1062–1064, 1973
123. Klagsbrun M: Human milk stimulates DNA synthesis and cellular proliferation in cultured fibroblasts. Proc Natl Acad Sci (USA) 75:5059–5061, 1978
124. Klagsbrun M, Neuman J, Tapper D: The mitogenic activity of human breast milk. J Surg Res 26:417–422, 1979
125. Laskowski M, Jr, Laskowski M: Crystalline trypsin inhibitor from colostrum. J Biol Chem 190:563–573, 1951
126. MacMahon B, Cole P, Lin TM, et al.: Age at first birth and breast cancer risk. Bull WHO 43:209–221, 1970
127. Conner AE: Elevated levels of sodium and chloride in milk from mastitic breast. Pediatrics 63:910–911, 1979
128. Hayes K, Danks DM, Gibas H, et al.: Cytomegalovirus in human milk. N Engl J Med 287:177–178, 1972
129. Stagno S, Reynolds DW, Alford CA: Breast feeding and the risk of cytomegalovirus (CMV) infection. Pediatr Res 13:469, 1979
130. Boxall EH, Flewett TH, Dane DS, et al.: Hepatitis-B surface antigen in breast milk. Lancet 2:1007–1008, 1974

131. Stevens CE, Beasley P, Tsui J, et al.: Vertical transmission of hepatitis B antigen in Taiwan. N Engl J Med 292:771–774, 1975
132. Buimovica-Klein E, Hite RL, Byrne T, et al.: Isolation of rubella virus in milk after postpartum immunization. J Pediatr 91:939–941, 1977
133. Dunkle LM, Schmidt RR, O'Conner DM: Neonatal herpes simplex infection possibly acquired via maternal breast milk. Pediatrics 63:250–251, 1979
134. Murray J, Murray AB: Breast milk and weights of Nigerian mothers and their infants. Am J Clin Nutr 32:737, 1979
135. Jelliffe DB, Jelliffe EFP: Lactation, conception, and the nutrition of the nursing mother and child. J Pediatr 81:829–833, 1972
136. Clarke TA, Markarian M, Griswold W, et al.: Hypernatremic dehydration resulting from inadequate breast-feeding. Pediatrics 63:931–932, 1979
137. Sarkar NH, Moore DH: On the possibility of a human breast cancer virus. Nature (Lond) 236:103–106, 1972
138. Forbes GB: Is human milk the best food for low birth weight babies? (Part 2.) Pediatr Res 12:434, 1978
139. Gross SJ, David RJ, Bouman L, et al.: Nutritional composition of human milk in mothers of preterm infants. Pediatr Res 13:400, 1979
140. Gross SJ, Wakil S, David RJ, et al.: Elevated immunoglobulin IgA in milk from mothers delivering preterm infants. Pediatr Res 13:449, 1979
141. Winfield CR, MacFaul R: Clinical study of prolonged jaundice in breast- and bottle-fed babies. Arch Dis Child 53:506–516, 1979
142. Luzeau R, Odjevre M, Levillain P, et al.: Activité de la lipoproteine lipase dans les laitz de femme inhibiteurs in vitro de la conjugaison de la bilirubine. Clin Chim Acta 59:133–138, 1975
143. Binder J, Johnson CF, Saboe B, et al.: Delayed elevation of serum phenylalanine level in a breast-fed child. Pediatrica 63:334–336, 1979
144. Lepow ML, Warren RJ, Gary N, et al.: Effect of sabin type I poliomyelitis vaccine administered by mouth to newborn infants. N Engl J Med 264:1071–1078, 1961
145. Warren RJ, Lepow ML, Bartsch GE, et al.: The relationship of maternal antibody, breast-feeding, and age to the susceptibility of newborn infants to infection with attenuated poliovirus. Pediatrics 34:4–13, 1964
146. Katz M, Plotkin SA: Oral polio immunization of the newborn infant: A possible method for overcoming interference by ingested antibodies. J Pediatr 73:267–270, 1968
147. American Academy of Pediatrics: Report of the Committee on Infectious Diseases (ed 13). Evanston, Ill., American Academy of Pediatrics, 1977, pp 3, 74
148. Talbot FB: Eczema in childhood. Med Clin North Am 1:985–996, 1918
149. Ratner B: A possible cause-factor of food allergy in certain infants. Am J Dis Child 36:277–288, 1928
150. Lyon GM: Allergy in an infant of three weeks. Am J Dis Child 36:1012–1016, 1928
151. Shannon WR: Demonstration of food proteins in human breast milk by anaphylactic experiments on guinea pigs. Am J Dis Child 22:223–231, 1921
152. Kuroume T, Oguri M, Matsumura T, et al.: Milk sensitivity and soybean sensitivity in the production of eczematous manifestations in breast-fed infants with particular reference to intrauterine sensitization. Ann Allergy 37:41–46, 1976
153. Fällström SP, Ahlstedt S, Hanson LÅ: Specific antibodies in infants with gastrointestinal intolerance to cow's milk protein. Int Arch Allergy Appl Immunol 56:97–105, 1978
154. Frick OL, German DF, Mills J: Development of allergy in children. I. Association with virus infections. J Allergy Clin Immunol 63:228–241, 1979
155. Gerrard JW: Allergy in breast fed babies to ingredients in breast milk. Ann Allergy 42:69–72, 1979

156. Illingworth RS: Abnormal substances excreted in human milk. Practitioner 171:533–538, 1953.
157. Gerrard JW, Lubos MC, Hardy LW, et al.: Milk allergy: Clinical picture and familial incidence. Can Med Assoc J 97:780–785, 1967
158. Kaplan MS, Solli NJ: Immunoglobulin E to cow's milk protein in breast-fed atopic children. J Allergy Clin Immunol 64:122–126, 1979
159. Jakabsson I, Lindberg T: Cow's milk as a cause of infantile colic in breast-fed infants. Lancet 2:437–439, 1978
160. Taj-Elden S: Favism in breast-fed infants. Arch Dis Child 46:121–123, 1971
161. Kattamis C: Favism in breast-fed infants. Arch Dis Child 46:741, 1971
162. Catz CS, Giacoia GP: Drugs and breast milk. Pediatr Clin North Am 19:151–166, 1972
163. Knowles JA: Breast milk: A source of more than nutrition for the neonate. Clin Toxicol 7:69–82, 1974
164. Wyckerheld-Bisdom CJ: Alcohol and nicotine poisoning in nurslings due to mother's milk Maandschr Kindergeneesk 6:332–341, 1937
165. Binkiewicz A, Robinson MJ, Senior B: Pseudo-Cushing syndrome caused by alcohol in breast milk. J Pediatr 93:965–967, 1978
166. Tyrala EE, Dodson WE: Caffeine secretion into breast milk. Arch Dis Child 54:787–800, 1979
167. Yurchak AM, Jusko WJ: Theophylline secretion into breast milk. Pediatrics 57:518–520, 1976
168. Knowles JA: Excretion of drugs in milk: A review. J Pediatr 66:1068–1082, 1965
169. Arena JM: Contamination of the ideal food. Nutr Today 5:2–8, 1970
170. O'Brien TE: Excretion of drugs in human milk. Am J Hosp Pharm 31:844–854, 1974
171. The Medical Letter: Update: Drugs in breast milk. Med Lett Drugs Therap 21:21–25, 1979
172. Wilson DJ, Locker DJ, Ritzen CA, et al.: DDT Concentrations in human milk. Am J Dis Child 125:814–817, 1973
173. Jukes TH: When friends or patients ask about DDT. JAMA 229:571–573, 1974
174. Olszyna-Marzys AE: Contaminants in human milk. Acta Paediatr Scand 67:571–576, 1978
175. Holdrinet MV, Braun HE, Frank P, et al.: Organochlorine residues in human adipose tissue and milk from Ontario residents, 1969–1974. Can J Public Health 68:74–80, 1977
176. Bakken AF, Seip M: Insecticides in human breast milk. Acta Paediatr Scand 65:535–539, 1976
177. Cam C: A new epidemic dermatosis of children. Ann Dermatol Syphiligr (Paris) 87:393–397, 1960
178. Amin-Zaki L, Elhassani S, Majeed MA, et al.: Studies on infants postnatally exposed to methylmercury. J Pediatr 85:81–84, 1974
179. Dyment PG, Hebertson LM, Decker WJ, et al.: Relationship between levels of chlorinated hydrocarbon insecticides in human milk and serum. Bull Environ Contam Toxicol 6:449–452, 1971
180. Miller RW: Pollutants in breast milk. J Pediatr 90:510–512, 1977
181. Department of National Health and Welfare: Polychlorinated Biphenyls. Committee Report, Information Letter DD-24. Ottawa, Department of National Health and Welfare, March 1978
182. Kuratsune M, Yoshimura T, Matsuzaka J, et al.: Epidemiologic study on Yusho, a poisoning caused by ingestion of rice oil contaminated with a commercial brand of polychlorinated biphenyls. Environ Health Perspect 1:119–128, 1972
183. Finebery L: PBBs: The ladies' milk is not for burning. J Pediatr 90:511–512, 1977
184. Widdowson EM: Protective properties of human milk and the effects of processing on them (Symposium Report). Arch Dis Child 53:684–686, 1978
185. Roy CC, Lescop J: Human milk banking: High rate of interest for a still uncertain credit balance. Am J Dis Child 133:255–256, 1979

186. Williamson S, Hewitt JH, Finucane E, et al.: Organization of bank of raw and pasteurised human milk for neonatal intensive care. Br Med J 1:393–396, 1978
187. Ford JE, Law BA, Marshall VME, et al.: Influence of the heat treatment of human milk on some of its protective constituents. J Pediatr 90:29–35, 1977
188. Raptopoulou-Gigi M, Marivick K, McClelland DBL: Antimicrobial proteins in sterilized human milk. Br Med J 1:12–14, 1977
189. Evans TJ, Ryley HC, Neale LM, et al.: Effect of storage and heat on antimicrobial proteins in human milk. Arch Dis Child 53:239–241, 1978
190. Liebhaber M, Lewiston NJ, Asquith MT, et al.: Alterations of lymphocytes and of antibody content of human milk after processing. J Pediatr 91:897–890, 1977
191. Eyres R, Elliott RB, Howie RN, et al.: Low-temperature pasteurisation of human milk. NZ Med J 87:134–135, 1978
192. Davidson DC, Poll RA, Roberts C: Bacteriological monitoring of unheated human milk. Arch Dis Child 54:760–764, 1979
193. Carroll L, Osman M, Davies DP, et al.: Bacteriological criteria for feeding raw breast-milk to babies on neonatal units. Lancet 2:732–733, 1979
194. Lucas A, Gibbs JAH, Lyster RLJ, et al.: Creamatocrit: Simple clinical technique for estimating fat concentration and energy value of human milk. Br Med J 1:1018–1020, 1978
195. Beer AE, Billingham RE: Immunologic benefits and hazards of milk in maternal-perinatal relationship. Ann Intern Med 83:865–871, 1975
196. Glaser J, Johnstone DE: Soybean milk as a substitute for mammalian milk in early infancy; with special reference to prevention of allergy to cow's milk. Ann Allergy 10:433–439, 1952
197. Johnstone DE, Glaser J: Use of soybean milk as an aid in prophylaxis of allergic disease in children. J Allergy 24:434–436, 1953
198. Brown EB, Josephson BM, Levine HS, et al.: A prospective study of allergy in a pediatric population. Am J Dis Child 117:693–698, 1969
199. Eastham EJ, Lichauco T, Grady MI: Antigenicity of infant formulas: Role of immature intestine on protein permeability. J Pediatr 93:561–564, 1978
200. Kjellman N-IM, Johansson SGO: Soy versus cow's milk in infants with a biparental history of atopic disease: Development of atopic disease and immunoglobulins from birth to 4 years of age. Clin Allergy 9:347–358, 1979
201. Applebaum RM: The modern management of successful breast-feeding. Pediatr Clin North Am 17:203–225, 1970
202. Applebaum RM: The obstetrician's approach to the breasts and breast-feeding. J Repr Med 14:98–116, 1975
203. Esterly NB: The obstetrician and breast feeding: Some views of women physicians. J Repr Med 14:89–97, 1975
204. La Leche: The Womanly Art of Breast Feeding (ed 2). Franklin Park, Ill., La Leche, 1963
205. Eiger M, Olds S: The complete Book of Breast Feeding. New York, Workman, 1972
206. Pryor K: Nursing Your Baby. New York, Harper & Row, 1975
207. Brewster DP: You Can Breastfeed Your Baby—Even in Special Situations. Emmaus, Pa., Rodale Press, 1979
208. Nunnally DM: A new approach in helping mothers breastfeed. JOGN Nurs 3:34–35, 1974
209. Bird IS: Breast-feeding classes on the post-partum unit. Am J Nurs 75:456, 1975
210. Sloper K, McKean L, Boum JD: Factors influencing breast-feeding. Arch Dis Child 50:165–170, 1975
211. Hill LF: A salute to La Leche League International. J Pediatr 73:161–162, 1968
212. Editorial: The infant-food industry. Lancet 2:503, 1976
213. Editorial: The infant-food industry. Lancet 1:1240–1241, 1978
214. Jelliffe DB, Jelliffe EFP: The infant food industry. Lancet 2:263, 1978
215. Baumslag N: Infant-food industry. Lancet 2:166, 1978

216. International Council of Infant Food Industries: Its aims and progress. Lancet 1:1250–1252, 1978
217. Jelliffe DB, Jelliffe EFP: Human Milk in the Modern World. Oxford, Oxford University Press, 1978, pp 408–413
218. Chopra JG: The role of Food and Drug Administration in food allergy. Ann Allergy 42:1–4, 1979
219. Bahna SL: Control of milk allergy: A challenge for physicians, mothers and industry. Ann Allergy 41:1–12, 1978

Appendix A
Milk-free Recipes

The recipes in this Appendix may be photocopied by the physician for patients' private use. Any other reproduction constitutes infringement on copyright.

Preparing meals free of cow's milk need not be difficult. Virtually every favorite recipe calling for milk can still be used by substituting for the milk an infant soybean formula or an easily purchased preparation such as Mocha Mix or another nondairy creamer. Children can thrive without any cow's milk. Milk-sensitive children in particular attain a new level of health and competence when milk is removed from their diets. Providing a milk-free diet is an exercise in creativity and can be fun. Delicious milk-free meals for the whole family are easily prepared by the interested homemaker. It is the same kind of test of one's ingenuity as is the art of good cooking of any type. There are endless recipes and formulations which can be prepared with milk substitutes or simply without milk. Some milk-sensitive subjects only require cow's milk that has been boiled (or canned evaporated milk).

All recipes presented in this appendix are free of cow's milk or its products, and many are also free of other common food allergens such as egg, wheat, and corn. Most of the recipes presented here have been adapted and modified from several sources. More recipes may be obtained from dietetic associations, certain food manufacturers, or books on allergy diets. A few sources are listed below:

1. Allergy Diets. Ralston Purina Company, Checkerboard Square, Saint Louis, Missouri 63199.
2. Baking for People with Food Allergies. Home and Garden Bulletin No. 147, U.S. Department of Agriculture, Superintendent of Documents, U.S. Government Printing Office, Washington, D.C. 20402.
3. Easy Appealing Recipes Using Pro-Sobee Soy Isolate Milk. Mead Johnson & Company, Evansville, Indiana 47721.
4. Tasty Recipes, Mull-Soy Liquid in Milk-Free Diets. Borden Inc., Pharmaceutical Products, 350 Madison Avenue, New York, N.Y. 10017.
5. Wheat-, Milk- and Egg-Free Recipes. Home Economics Department, The Quaker Oats Company, Merchandise Mart Plaza, Chicago, Illinois 60611.

Table 1
Beverages

Pure fruit juices

Juices of fruits such as apple, orange, grapefruit, grape, apricot, peach, pear nectar, guana, mango, etc., are excellent and easy-to-prepare beverages for the milk-sensitive subject.

Pure vegetable juices

Vegetables such as tomatoes, carrots, and beets are also good beverages.

Beverages containing soy formula

Hawaiian Fling. Mix equal parts of pineapple juice and soybean formula. Add 1 teaspoon sugar per cup of mixture or according to taste. Mix well and chill.

Apricot Dream. Equal parts of apricot nectar and soybean formula. May be sweetened as desired with sugar per cup of mixture. Mix well and chill.

Banana-Honey Flip. 1 cup soybean formula, 1 ripe banana, and 1 tablespoon honey. Mix in a blender or mash well with a fork and stir.

Apricot Shake. ¼ cup soybean formula, ¼ cup cold water, ½ cup finely cracked ice, and ½ cup sieved, sweetened, stewed apricots.

Combine all ingredients in a shaker or jar with a tight-fitting lid. Cover container and shake well. Serve at once.

Banana shake. 1 ripe banana, 2 tablespoons sugar, ½ cup soybean formula, ½ cup cold water, and finely cracked ice.

Peel and slice banana; beat with rotary or electric beater or in electric blender until smooth and creamy. Beat in sugar. Add soybean formula and water; beat until well blended. Pour into ice-filled glasses and serve at once.

Orange Frost. ¼ cup soybean formula, ¼ cup cold water, ½ cup orange juice, 1 tablespoon sugar, 1 teaspoon lemon juice, and ½ cup cracked ice.

Combine all ingredients in a shaker or jar with a tight-fitting lid. Cover container and shake well. Serve at once. Makes 1¼ cups.

Table 2
Main Dishes

Fish Chowder. 3 tablespoons finely chopped onion, 1 tablespoon all-vegetable margarine, 4 cups hot water, 1 teaspoon salt, ¼ teaspoon pepper, 1½ cups diced, pared potatoes, ½ cup diced carrots, and 1½ cups flaked fish, cooked or canned.

Cook onion slowly in hot all-vegetable margarine. Add water and seasonings. Heat to boiling. Add vegetables. Cook 25 minutes or until tender. Add fish and heat thoroughly. Yields 4 servings.

Meat Loaf. ½ lb ground chuck, ¼ cup soybean formula, ¼ cup uncooked oatmeal, 1 tablespoon grated carrot, 1 tablespoon finely chopped onion, and salt and pepper to taste.

Mix all ingredients thoroughly. Shape into loaf. Bake at 350°F (175°C) for 30 minutes.

Chicken Fricassee. Cut into serving pieces ½ frying chicken. Roll in rice or wheat flour, salt and pepper mixture. Brown chicken pieces in 2 tablespoons all-vegetable margarine in skillet. Place in baking dish.

Prepare medium cream sauce with rye or rice flour. (see p 182). Pour sauce over chicken. Sprinkle top with crushed potato chips. Bake at 350°F (175°C) for 1 hour.

Ham-Potato Casserole. Arrange in alternate layers in greased baking dish: 1 cup diced baked ham, and 2 medium potatoes, pared and thinly sliced.

Make thin white sauce with: 1 tablespoon all-vegetable margarine, 1 tablespoon rice flour, and 1¼ cups soybean formula.

Add: ½ small chopped onion, and 1 tablespoon chopped green pepper. Black pepper and a dash of garlic salt may be added if desired.

Pour mixture over the potatoes and ham. With a fork gently lift potatoes and ham so sauce reaches the bottom of the dish. Bake at 400°F (200°C) on center rack of oven about 1 hour, or until potatoes are tender when pierced with a fork. Yields 2 servings.

Tuna Casserole. Mix and heat to boiling: ½ cup soybean formula and 1½ tablespoons cornstarch.

Continue stirring until thickened, if sauce seems too thick, add a little more water.

Remove sauce from heat and add: 1 teaspoon minced onion, ¼ teaspoon celery salt, dash of garlic salt, and ½ can tuna, broken into pieces.

Stir in lightly: ⅓ cup canned or fresh peas, and 1 cup of lightly crushed potato chips (save a few chips for top of casserole).

Pour into greased baking dish and garnish with crushed potato chips. Bake at 400°F (200°C) on center rack of oven for 30 or 40 minutes, or until bubbly and brown on top.

Lamb Stew. ½ lb cut-up lamb, 1 tablespoon rice flour, ¾ teaspoon salt, 1 tablespoon lamb drippings or other milk-free fat, 1¼ cups hot water, 1½ cups diced, pared sweet potatoes, and 1 tablespoon rice flour.

Roll lamb in mixture of flour and salt. Bron in hot fat. Add water. Cover; simmer for 1 hour. Add potatoes; cover and cook 25 minutes longer, or until tender. Make gravy with liquid and 1 tablespoon rice flour. Yields 3 servings.

Lamb with Rice. 3 tablespoons rice flour, 2 tablespoons lamb drippings or other milk-free fat, 1 cup hot water, ½ teaspoon salt, 1 cup diced lamb, and 1½ cups hot cooked rice.

Brown rice flour in fat. Add water and salt. Cook and stir until thick and smooth. Add lamb and heat thoroughly. Serve over rice. Yields 3 servings.

Braised Lamb Shank. 2 lamb shanks, ½ teaspoon salt, 2 tablespoons hot lamb drippings or other milk-free fat, ¾ cup hot water, 2 tablespoons rice flour, and 2 tablespoons cold water.

Sprinkle meat with salt. In heavy pan with tight-fitting cover, brown meat in fat. Add hot water, and cover. Simmer 1 hour, or until tender, adding more water if necessary. Remove meat to hot platter. Mix flour and water until smooth. Add to liquid in pan, stirring until thickened. Yields 2 servings.

Lamb Loaf. ½ lb ground lamb, ½ teaspoon salt, ½ cup cranberry juice, and ¼ cup rye cracker crumbs.

Combine all ingredients. Pack into loaf pan. Bake at 350°F (160°C) for 1 hour. Yields 4 servings.

Lamb Liver Slices With Spiced Prune Sauce. ⅔ cup dried prunes, 1½ cups water, ¼ cup sugar, ½ teaspoon citric acid crystals, 1 tablespoon rice flour, 1 lb sliced lamb liver, 1 teaspoon salt, and 2 tablespoons lamb drippings or other fat.

Cover prunes with water and simmer until tender. Drain and cut up prunes, reserving liquid. Combine sugar, citric acid crystals, and rice flour. Gradually stir in liquids from prunes (about ½ cup). Cook and stir until slightly thickened. Add cut up prunes and heat thoroughly. Sprinkle liver with salt. Brown on both sides in fat (about 2 minutes on each side). Serve with prune sauce. Yields 4 servings.

Table 3
Vegetables

Mashed Potatoes. 2 medium-sized potatoes, pared and quartered, and 1 cup water.

Boil potatoes in a covered pan about 20 minutes or until tender. Drain off water and mash potatoes well. Beat in heated soybean formula gradually until potatoes are light and fluffy. Parsley or a dash of paprika can be added for flavor and looks.

Beets-Harvard. 2 tablespoons sugar, ¼ teaspoon salt, ½ teaspoon citric acid crystals, 1 tablespoon rice flour, ½ cup beet liquid or water, and 1 cup hot, sliced or diced cooked beets.

Combine sugar, salt, citric acid crystals and flour. Stir in water. Cook and stir until thickened (about 2 minutes). Add beets and heat thoroughly. Yields 2 servings.

Pickled Beets-Harvard. Omit rice flour in above recipe. Increase citric acid to 1 teaspoon. Combine sugar, salt, citric acid crystals and water. Pour over beets. Chill.

Sweet Potatoes—Glazed. Put whole or split, cooked, pared sweet potatoes in saucepan. For each medium-sized potato, add 1 tablespoon lamb drippings or other fat, 2 tablespoons sugar. Cook over low heat, turning frequently, until thoroughly heated and coated with sugar mixture.

Sweet Potato Balls. Mash cooked sweet potatoes with lamb drippings or other fat and salt to taste. Shape into balls. Roll in rye cracker crumbs. Put in shallow greased baking dish. Heat thoroughly in oven at 375°F (190°C).

Lima Bean or Split Pea Soup. 1 cup split peas or lima beans, 2 tablespoons bacon fat, diced crisp bacon, 1 quart water, and salt.

Cook peas or beans with salt to a smooth puree. Add bacon and bacon fat before serving.

Table 4
Salad Dressings

Basic Dressing. 2 tablespoons rice flour, ½ teaspoon salt, 2 tablespoons sugar, 1 teaspoon citric acid crystals, ½ cup water, ½ cup cooking oil, and ¼ cup Caramel Sugar Syrup.

Mix together dry ingredients. Stir in water. Cook, stirring, over low heat 2 minutes, or until thickened. Cool. With rotary beater, beat in oil a tablespoon at a time. Beat in syrup. Yields 1 cup.

Caramel sugar syrup: Put ¼ cup sugar into small skillet over low heat. Stir until sugar melts and turns golden brown. Add ¾ cup sugar and 1 cup boiling water. Cook until smooth, stirring constantly. Boil 10 minutes longer without stirring. Yields ¾ cup.

Olive Dressing. Add ¼ cup finely cut ripe olives to above basic dressing. Serve on spinach or sweet potato salad.

Cranberry Dressing. Add ¼ cup cranberry juice to above basic dressing. Serve on spinach salad.

Table 5
Salads

Beets. Cut up ½ cup cold, cooked beets. Pour over them 2 tablespoons basic dressing. Sprinkle with 2 tablespoons rye cracker crumbs.

Spinach. Rinse and tear up enough fresh spinach to make 1 cup. Chill. Pour over it 2 tablespoons basic, olive, or cranberry dressing. Sprinkle with 2 tablespoons rye cracker crumbs.

Sweet Potato. Cut up ½ cup cold, cooked sweet potatoes. Pour over them 2 tablespoons basic or olive dressing. Sprinkle with 2 tablespoons rye cracker crumbs.

Table 6
Gravies and Sauces

Rice Flour Gravy.   Heat 3 tablespoons fat in a frying pan. Add 2 tablespoons rice flour and brown while stirring. Slowly add 1¼ cups soybean formula; stir constantly to keep smooth. Cook on low heat until thick and smooth, stirring frequently. Add salt and pepper to taste.

Rye Flour Gravy.   Heat 3 tablespoons fat in a frying pan. Add 2 tablespoons rye flour and brown while stirring. Slowly add ¾ cup soybean formula; stir constantly to keep smooth. Cook on low heat until thick and smooth, stirring frequently. Add salt and pepper to taste.

Medium Cream Sauce with Rye Flour.   Melt 2 tablespoons all-vegetable margarine in a 1-quart saucepan. Add 2 tablespoons rye flour and stir until smooth. Add ¾ cup soybean formula and cook until smooth, stirring constantly. Add salt and pepper to taste.

Medium Cream Sauce with Rice Flour.   Melt 2 tablespoons all-vegetable margarine in a 1-quart saucepan. Add 2 tablespoons rice flour and stir. Add 1¼ cups soybean formula and cook until smooth, stirring constantly. Add salt and pepper to taste.

Appendixes

Table 7
Cookies

Herb Crisps. Spread 12 rye crackers lightly with herb spread (2 tablespoons all-vegetable margarine plus ½ teaspoon basil, thyme, ginger or celery salt). Place on rack in shallow pan. Toast in oven at 350°F (175°C) for 5 minutes. Serve warm or cold.

Cinnamon Crisps. 12 rye crackers, 2 tablespoons all-vegetable margarine, 2 tablespoons sugar, 1 teaspoon cinnamon.
Spread crackers with all-vegetable margarine. Sprinkle with sugar-cinnamon mixture. Bake 5 minutes at 400°F (200°C). Serve warm or cold.

Date Bars. 3 eggs, ⅔ cup brown sugar, firmly packed, 1 cup rye cracker crumbs, 1¼ cups finely chopped dates, ¾ cup chopped nuts.
Beat eggs until thick and foamy. Add brown sugar gradually. Beat after each addition. Beat in cracker crumbs, dates, and nuts. Mix thoroughly. Pour into buttered 8-inch-square pan. Bake at 325°F (160°C) for 35–40 minutes or until firm to the touch. Loosen sides with knife. Let stand 15 minutes before cutting. Yields 15 bars (1½ × 2 in).

Butterscotch Brownies. ¼ cup all-vegetable shortening, 1 cup light brown sugar (firmly packed), 1 egg, ¾ cup all-purpose wheat flour, 1 teaspoon baking powder, ½ teaspoon vanilla.
Melt shortening over low heat. Remove from heat and blend in brown sugar. Let cool. Stir in egg. Sift together and stir in flour and baking powder. Stir in vanilla. Spread in well-greased and floured 8-inch-square pan. Bake at 350°F (175°C) for 20–25 minutes, until a light touch with finger leaves slight imprint. Cut into bars while warm. Makes 18 bars (1 × 2½ inches).

Sugar Cookies. 2 eggs, ⅔ cup cooking oil, 2 teaspoons vanilla, 1 teaspoon grated lemon rind, ¾ cup sugar, 2 cups sifted all-purpose flour, 2 teaspoons baking powder, ½ teaspoon salt.
Heat oven to 400°F. Beat eggs with fork until well blended. Stir in oil, vanilla, lemon rind. Blend in sugar until mixture thickens. Sift together flour, baking powder, salt, and stir into oil mixture. Drop with teaspoon 2 inches apart on ungreased baking sheet. Flatten with bottom of greased drinking glass dipped in sugar. Bake at 400°F (200°C) for 10 minutes or until a delicate brown. Yields about 3 dozen cookies.

Molasses Cookies. Cream together until light and fluffy: 1 cup all-vegetable margarine, ½ cup granulated sugar, ½ cup brown sugar, 1 teaspoon baking powder, ½ teaspoon baking soda, 2 teaspoons vanilla. Add to this mixture: ½ cup molasses. Add and mix well: ¼ cup cornstarch. Add and mix: ½ cup soybean formula. Stir in gradually: 3 cups sifted rye flour. When flour is thoroughly mixed, add: 1 cup raisins, 1 cup chopped nuts.
Chill dough for about 30 minutes. Shape dough into balls the size of a walnut and bake on a greased cookie sheet at 400°F (200°C) for 7–10 minutes or until light brown. Yields approximately 8 dozen cookies.
Note: Honey may be substituted for molasses to make honey cookies.

Raisin Oatmeal Cookies. Cream together until light and fluffy: 1 cup all-vegetable margarine, ½ cup sugar, 1 cup light brown sugar, 2 teaspoons cinnamon, ½ teaspoon mace. Add to first mixture: ⅓ cup soybean formula, 2 tablespoons cornstarch, 1 teaspoon baking powder. Beat well and add: ⅓ cup soybean formula, 2 cups sifted rye flour. Add and mix well: 2 cups oatmeal, 1 cup raisins, ¾ cup chopped dates, 1 cup chopped walnuts.

If dough seems too stiff, add a little more soybean formula. Chill dough. Shape dough into balls about the size of a walnut. Bake on a greased cookie sheet at 375°F (190°C) for 15 minutes or until light brown.

Snowballs. Mix until smooth and creamy: 1 cup all-vegetable margarine, 1 cup powdered sugar, packed, 2 teaspoons vanilla. Add and mix well: ½ cup soybean formula, ¼ cup cornstarch. Gradually beat in: 2½ cups sifted rice flour. Add: 1 cup chopped pecans, ⅔ cup chopped walnuts.

Chill dough. Shape dough in rough balls the size of a walnut and decorate with pieces of maraschino cherries or colored pineapple. Bake at 350°F (175°C) 20–30 minutes on ungreased cookie sheet. Roll balls in powdered sugar while they are still warm.

Chocolate Fudge. Mix in a large saucepan: 2 cups sugar, 2 tablespoons cocoa, ¼ cup corn syrup. Add and mix until smooth: ½ cup soybean formula.

Cook over moderate heat, stirring frequently, until a soft ball forms in cold water or the mixture registers 230°F on a candy thermometer. Remove from heat and add: 2 tablespoons all-vegetable margarine, 1 teaspoon vanilla. Beat until candy starts to turn dull; then pour into a greased dish. Cut when firm.

Table 8
Desserts

Baked Custard. 1 cup water, 1 tablespoon Cream of Rice, dash salt, 2 tablespoons sugar, 2 egg yolks, ¼ teaspoon vanilla, nutmeg.

Bring water to boil. Sprinkle in Cream of Rice and cook, stirring constantly until slightly thickened. Lower heat; cover and simmer 5 minutes. Remove from heat and beat vigorously with rotary beater for 2 minutes. Add salt and 1 tablespoon sugar. Beat egg yolks with remaining tablespoon sugar. Gradually beat in rice mixture. Stir in vanilla. Strain through fine sieve. Pour into 2 small custard cups and sprinkle with grated nutmeg. Place in pan of hot water. Bake in preheated 325°F (160°C) oven for 50 minutes or until barely set.

If an electric blender is used, blend rice mixture until smooth, about 2 minutes. Add remaining ingredients and blend again. It is not necessary to strain this mixture. Finish as directed above.

Apricot Rice Pudding. 1 tablespoon uncooked rice, ¾ cup hot water, ¼ cup soybean formula, pinch of salt, 2 tablespoons brown sugar, ¼ cup strained, stewed apricot, ¼ teaspoon vanilla.

Wash rice and put in 1-pint baking dish. Add water, soybean formula, salt and sugar, and blend well. Bake at 325°F (160°C) for 1½ hours, stirring once in awhile. Remove from oven and stir in strained apricot. Return to oven and continue baking for ½ hour longer. Remove from oven and stir in vanilla. Cool at room temperature and then chill in refrigerator. Serve cold. Yields 1 serving.

Butterscotch Pudding. Mix thoroughly: 1 cup brown sugar, 4 tablespoons cornstarch, ½ teaspoon salt.

Add and beat until smooth: 1 cup soybean formula, 2 teaspoons vanilla. Add gradually 1 cup soybean formula.

Cook over low heat, stirring constantly, until thick. Remove from heat and add 2 tablespoons all-vegetable margarine.

Cornstarch Pudding. 1 cup fruit juice (orange, pineapple, or grape), 1 cup water, ¼ cup sugar, 3 tablespoons cornstarch.

Mix cornstarch with sugar and blend with a small amount of the water into a paste. Add the paste to the rest of the water. Stir in the fruit juice. Cook directly over low heat, stirring constantly until thick. Yields four ½-cup servings.

Fruit Tapioca. Follow the recipe for cornstarch pudding, but substitute 4 tablespoons quick-cooking tapioca for cornstarch. Combine ingredients and cook in the top of a double boiler, over boiling water, about 20 minutes (until the tapioca is transparent).

Apple Tapioca. 1½ cups boiling water, 1½ tablespoons quick-cooking tapioca, 4 medium apples, ⅓ cup sugar, ⅛ teaspoon salt.

Add the tapioca, sugar, and salt to the boiling water in the top of a double boiler. Cook over boiling water until transparent (about 20 minutes). Pare and core the apples; arrange in a greased baking dish. Pour the tapioca over and around the apples. Bake at 375°F (190°C) until the apples are tender. Serve warm or cold.

Frozen Delight. 1 cup soybean formula, 3 tablespoons sugar, 1 teaspoon unflavored gelatin, 1 tablespoon water, 1 teaspoon vanilla.

Chill soybean formula; add sugar and beat with a rotary beater or electric mixer until sugar is dissolved. Soften gelatin in water for 3 minutes. Place over hot water and stir until gelatin is dissolved. Stir into soybean formula mixture. Add vanilla. Pour into freezing tray. Cover tray with waxed paper. Freeze to a firm mush. Remove waxed paper and pour into chilled bowl. Beat with rotary beater or electric mixer until fluffy but not melted. Quickly return to freezer. Freeze until firm. Yields about 2 cups.

Spice Cake with Pineapple Icing. Cream together: ½ cup sugar, ¼ cup all-vegetable margarine, add 1 cup soybean formula. Gradually add mixture of: ½ teaspoon cinnamon, ½ teaspoon mace, ¼ teaspoon salt, ½ teaspoon baking soda, ½ teaspoon baking powder, ¼ cup cornstarch, 1 cup sifted rye flour. Beat well. Add: 1 teaspoon vanilla. Pour into 8-inch cake pan. Bake at 375°F (190°C) for 25–30 minutes.

Pineapple Icing. Cream well: 1 tablespoon all-vegetable margarine, 2 cups powdered sugar, 2 tablespoons well-drained crushed pineapple, ½ teaspoon vanilla.

Brown Sugar Spice Cake. Cream together: ½ cup all-vegetable margarine, ½ cup sugar, ½ cup brown sugar, ½ teaspoon salt, 1 teaspoon cinnamon, ½ teaspoon mace, 1 teaspoon vanilla. Add: 1 teaspoon baking soda, 1 teaspoon baking powder. Add alternately beginning and ending with flour: 1¼ cup soybean formula, 2 cups sifted rice flour (save a small portion of the flour to mix with raisins)

Stir in: ½ cup raisins, ½ cup chopped nuts. Bake in a well-greased, 9-inch cake pan for about 30 minutes. Sprinkle with powdered sugar when cold.

Rice Ring With Fruit. 3 cups pineapple juice, 1 cup strawberries, 1 banana, 1 peach, 2 tablespoons sugar, ½ teaspoon salt, ¾ cup Cream of Rice.

Place pineapple juice, sugar, and salt in saucepan and bring to a boil. Sprinkle in Cream of Rice and cook, stirring constantly until slightly thickened. Lower heat; cover and simmer 5 minutes. Stir well and pour into lightly oiled 3-cup ring mold. Cover tightly with waxed paper or aluminum foil and chill until firm. Just before serving, unmold on cold platter and fill center with sliced strawberries, bananas, and peaches. Serve with lemon sauce. Yields 6 servings.

Lemon Sherbet. Sprinkle 1 tablespoon unflavored gelatin on ½ cup water. Place over low heat and stir until gelatin is dissolved. Put into a 2-quart bowl: 4 cups soybean formula, ½ cup lemon juice, 1 cup sugar, 1 teaspoon grated lemon rind.

Mix ingredients until all sugar is dissolved. Add gelatin mixture. Place mixture in freezer trays. When partially frozen, beat until smooth but not melted, and freeze until firm.

Orange Sherbet. Follow directions for making gelatin mixture in lemon sherbet recipe. Add 1½ cups cold water. Put into a 3-quart bowl: 1½ cups sugar, 2 cups orange juice, 3 tablespoons lemon juice, 2 cups soybean formula, grated rind of 1 orange.

Follow same procedure as with lemon sherbet.

Milk-free Ice Cream. Chill bowls and beaters. Beat 4 eggs until thick and cream-colored. Add ¼ cup sugar and ½ teaspoon vanilla. Beat again. Beat 2 cups nondairy dessert topping. Fold into eggs with spatula. Freeze until almost frozen. Re-beat and freeze again.

Soybean Formula Ice Cream. Sprinkle 1 tablespoon unflavored gelatin on ½ cup water. Place over low heat and stir until gelatin is dissolved. Add 1 cup water. Then add: 1 cup soybean formula, 2 cups fresh strawberries and ½ cup sugar (or 1 package frozen strawberries).

Beat and turn into freezer tray. When partially frozen, beat until smooth but not melted and freeze until firm.

Coffee, vanilla, chocolate, and peppermint flavors may be made. Add to basic soybean formula and gelatin mixture. Add flavoring and sugar to taste. Beat and proceed as above.

Banana-base Ice Cream, Sherbets, Shakes, Slushes. Banana base is simple to make and convenient to use for individual servings of many frozen desserts. The innovative homemaker can add a wide variety of healthful and tasty fruits.

Ripe bananas—as many as desired—and orange juice, one ounce per banana.

Blend peeled bananas with orange juice. Pour into empty plastic ice cream container. Place in freezer. After well frozen, pour beverage of your choice over the frozen bananas. Use ½ cup of beverage to make 1 cup of ice cream. With large spoon, scrape off in layers the frozen banana, rotating the container so the remaining frozen banana has a smooth surface. Soon there will be a soft slush. Scraping more banana off will produce a thicker dessert. Stir in same container with bottom of spoon to make creamy smooth consistency. Place in dish and eat as is or cover with your favorite fresh fruit or nuts.

For banana-base shakes or ice cream, use mocha mix or soybean infant formula as the beverage. For slushes, use your favorite fruit juice. For sherbets, do as for slushes but scrape off more frozen banana to increase thickness. Use your imagination. Mix in fresh fruits in season. If you do not like orange juice, use lemonade or limeade. If citrus fruits disagree with you, use other fruit juices. If you prefer just bananas, add 1 teaspoon honey per banana to sweeten if desired.

Each child can mix his own favorite milk-free ice cream. The product, with a little experience and experimentation, can be superior to any commercial ice cream in taste, nutritional value, and appeal. Make your own milk-free ice cream cones.

Fruited Gelatin. ¾ cup dried fruit, 3 cups water, 1 tablespoon unflavored gelatin, ¼ cup cold water, ½ teaspoon citric acid crystals, ⅔ cup sugar.

Cook fruit in three cups water for 30 minutes or until tender. Drain, saving juice. Add water to make 1¾ cups. Soften gelatin in ¼ cup cold water. Heat juice, citric acid, and sugar to boiling. Add gelatin, stirring until dissolved. Chill. When beginning to thicken, cut up fruit and add. Rinse mold with water. Pour in gelatin mixture. Chill until firm. Yields 4 servings.

Dried apricots, peaches, pitted prunes, or a mixture of these can be used. 2 cups fresh sliced peaches can be used if the cooking time is decreased to 15 minutes.

Fruit Betty. 6 rye crackers, crumbled, 1 cup cooked dried fruit, drained and cut up, ¼ teaspoon citric acid crystals, ½ cup fruit juice, 1 tablespoon sugar.

Arrange in greased baking dish layers of fruit and cracker crumbs, fruit on bottom, crumbs on top. Stir citric acid into juice and pour over fruit and crumbs. Sprinkle with sugar. Bake at 375°F (190°C) for 30 minutes. Serve warm or cold. Yields 2 servings.

For Fruit and Juice: Cook ⅔ cup dried fruit in 1¼ cups water until tender. To apricots, add ½ cup sugar; to prunes or peaches, add ⅓ cup sugar. Cook 5 minutes longer.

Tapioca Pudding. 1 cup hot water, 2-⅓ tablespoons quick-cooking tapioca, ¼ cup sugar, ⅛ teaspoon salt, ¼ teaspoon vanilla.

Combine water, tapioca, sugar, and salt. Cook and stir over medium heat until clear and mixture starts to boil (about 5 minutes). Cool. Add vanilla. Chill. Yields 2 servings.

Peach: Before chilling the above, add ½ cup drained cooked, fresh or dried, cut-up peaches.

Appendix B

Reference Tables on the Composition of Human Milk, Cow's Milk, Goat's Milk, and a Variety of Proprietary Formulas

Table 1
Composition of Human and Cow's Milks

Milk Constitutent	Unit	Human Range	Human Average	Cow's Range	Cow's Average
Water	gm/dl	87–89	87.6	87–88	87.3
Protein	gm/dl	0.7 – 2.0	1.2	2.8 – 4.1	3.3
Lactose	gm/dl	6.5 – 7.0	7.0	4.5 – 5.0	4.8
Fat	gm/dl	3.5 – 5.0	3.8	3.1 – 5.2	3.7
Minerals	gm/dl	0.16– 0.27	0.21	0.64– 0.75	0.72
Calories	kcal/oz	18–24	20	17–25	20
Osmolarity	mOsm/liter		273		260
Renal solute load	mOsm/liter	75–80	79	221–230	226
Minerals					
Sodium	mEq/liter	2–13	7	13.5 –93	25
Potassium	mEq/liter	9.5 –17.5	14	9.7 –74	35
Chloride	mEq/liter	2.6 –21	12	27–40	29
Calcium	mg/liter	170–610	340	560–3810	1240
Phosphorus	mg/liter	70–270	140	560–1120	950

Sulphur	mg/liter	50–300	140	240–360	300
Magnesium	mg/liter	20–60	40	70–220	120
Iron	mg/liter	0.5 – 1.8	1.5	0.2 – 2.0	1.0
Zinc	mg/liter	0.17– 3.0	1.2	1.9 – 6.6	3.8
Copper	mg/liter	0.1 – 0.7	0.4	0.2 – 0.8	0.3
Iodine	mg/liter	0.03– 0.09	0.07	0.13– 1.8	0.21
Vitamins					
Vitamin A	IU/liter	600–5000	1898	800–2500	1025
Vitamin D	IU/liter	20–100	22	5–40	14
Vitamin E	IU/liter	6–7	6.6	0.4 – 1.5	1.0
Vitamin C	mg/liter	12–108	43	9–20	16
Thiamine (B_1)	mcg/liter	100–360	200	300–440	350
Riboflavin (B_2)	mcg/liter	150–800	370	1000–2600	1750
Pyridoxin (B_6)	mcg/liter	100–110	105	480–640	500
Niacin	mcg/liter	660–3300	1470	850–1000	950
Pantothenate	mcg/liter	1840–2200	2000	3300–3460	3400
Vitamin B_{12}	mcg/liter	0.3 – 0.35	0.34	4– 5.6	5.3

Data collected from several sources and based on mature milk

Table 2
Amino Acids in Human and Cow's Milks

Amino Acid (mg/liter)	Human Range	Human Average	Cow's Range	Cow's Average
Essential				
Histidine	160–340	230	680–1300	950
Isoleucine	460–1020	860	1840–2900	2280
Leucine	720–1610	1280	2400–5420	3560
Lysine	530–1040	790	2200–3100	2570
Methionine	180–250	230	600–1090	870
Phenylalanine	300–640	480	1400–2200	1720
Threonine	400–760	620	1200–2200	1640
Tryptophan	130–260	220	400–800	500
Valine	480–1140	800	1890–2800	2450
Nonessential				
Arginine	370–510	450	1240–1370	1290
Alanine	200–350	300	750–1250	800
Aspartic acid	620–1260	1160	1660–2550	1920
Cystine	200–290	220	290–350	320
Glutamic acid	1500–2800	2300	6300–7440	6500
Glycine	0	0		110
Proline	560–900	800	2500–3180	2520
Serine		690	1600–1850	1640
Tyrosine	450–620	610	1790–1900	1840

Data collected from several sources and based on mature milk

Table 3
Fatty Acids in Human and Cow's Milks

Fatty Acid (% of total)	Human Range	Human Average	Cow's Range	Cow's Average
Essential				
Linoleic		10.6		2.1
Nonessential unsaturated				
Oleic	36.4–39.5	37.4	17.7–32.2	29.6
Palmitoleic		3.4		3.2
Linolenic		Trace		
Nonessential saturated				
Palmitic	21.6–26.7	23.2	25.3–36.6	26.3
Stearic	6.8–9.0	7.7	8.1–13.2	9.2
Myristic	6.6–8.6	7.9	10.5–12.1	11.8
Lauric	4.7–6.4	5.8	2.2–3.7	3.6
Capric	0.8–2.2	1.7	2.6–3.2	2.9
Caprylic	0.1–0.4	0.3	1.2–1.5	1.3
Caproic		0.1	1.0–2.0	1.4
Butyric	0.3–0.4	0.4	2.7–3.1	3.0

Data collected from several sources and based on mature milk

Table 4
Nutritional Constituents of Human Milk, Commercial Cow's Milk, Goat's Milk, and Some Preparations of Standard Cow's Milk Formulas

Name of Product (Manufacturer)	Calories kcal/oz	Calories kcal/dl	Protein gm/dl	Fat gm/dl	Carbohydrate gm/dl	Na mEq/liter	K mEq/liter	Cl mEq/liter	Ca mg/liter	P mg/liter	Fe mg/liter	Vit A IU/liter	Vit D IU/liter	Vit E IU/liter	Vit C mg/liter	Thiamine μg/liter	Niacin μg/liter	Pyridoxine μg/liter	Pantothenate μg/liter	Riboflavin μg/liter
HUMAN MILK	20	68	1.2	3.8	7.0	7	14	12	340	140	1.5	1898	22	6.6	43	200	1470	105	2000	370
COW'S MILK, FORTIFIED	20	68	3.3	3.7	4.8	25	35	29	1240	950	1	1025	414	1	16	350	950	500	3400	1750
GOAT'S MILK																				
Fresh	21	71	3.6	4.0	4.6	14	46	45	1280	1049	5	2074	24		15	400	3300	70	3400	1840
Powder (Dales, Cutter)	20	68	3.3	4.1	4.7	18	46	45	1220	1100	Trace				14	480	2700	70	2900	1140
STANDARD COW'S MILK FORMULAS																				
Bremil, with Fe (Borden)	20	68	1.5	3.5	7.0	11	16	13	700	360	8.5	2640	423	5.3	53	420	6340	420		1060
Bremil Powder, with Fe (Borden)	20	68	1.5	3.5	7.1	16	36	13	700	360	8.5	2640	423	5.3	53	420	6340	420		1060
Enfamil† (Mead-Johnson)	20	68	1.5	3.7	7.0	12	19	12	640	500	1.5	1600	423	12	53	423	8000	400	3000	660
Infant Formula (Baker)	20	68	2.2	3.3	7.0	17	23	19	840	740	7.9	1782	423		35	446	7400	297		1102
Lactogen Powder (Nestlé)	20	68	2.4	3.5	7.6	13	27	17	840	740	7									
Lactogen Powder, Full Protein (Nestlé)	20	68	3.4	2.9	7.9	19	38	24	1220	1060	7									
Modilac (Gerber)	20	68	2.2	2.7	7.8	17	27	19	840	740	10.6	1585	423		48	528	5300	740		740
Nan Powder (Nestlé)	20	68	1.6	3.4	7.3	10	19	12	440	460	7									
Pelargon Powder (Nestlé)	22	74	2.8	2.9	9.7	16	32	20	1040	900	7									
Similac† (Ross)	20	68	1.6	3.6	7.2	11	20	15	510	390	Trace	2500	400	15	55	650	7000	400	3000	1000
SMA S-26 (Wyeth)	20	68	1.5	3.6	7.2	7	14	11	462	343	13	2650	440	9.9	60	737	1045	440	2200	1100
EVAPORATED COW'S MILK	21	71	3.8	4.0	5.4	28	39	32	1346	1025	1	1850	420	1.3	5.5	280	1000	370	3500	1900

*Blank space indicates that the information could not be obtained

†Also available with iron supplement

Table 5
Nutritional Constituents of Some Hypoallergenic Infant Formulas

Name of Product (Manufacturer)	Calories kcal/oz	Calories kcal/dl	Protein Type	Protein gm/dl	Fat Type	Fat gm/dl	Carbohydrate Type	Carbohydrate gm/dl	Na mEq/liter	K mEq/liter	Cl mEq/liter	Ca mg/liter	P mg/liter	Fe mg/liter	Vit A IU/liter	Vit D IU/liter	Vit E IU/liter	Vit C mg/liter	Thiamine μ/liter	Niacin μ/liter	Pyridoxine μ/liter	Pantothenate μ/liter	Riboflavin μ/liter
SOYBEAN FORMULAS																							
Isomil (Ross)	20	68	Soy isolate	2.0	Corn, Coconut	3.6	Sucrose, Maltodextrins	6.8	13	18	15	700	500	12	2500	400	15	55	400	6000	400	5000	600
Mull-Soy Liquid (Borden)	20	68	Soy	3.1	Soy oil	3.6	Sucrose, Inverted sucrose	5.2	16	40	16	1200	920	5	2100	423	10.6	42	530	9500	420	1000	845
Neo-Mull-Soy (Syntex)	20	68	Soy isolate	1.8	Soy oil	3.6	Sucrose	6.6	17	25	6	880	660	11	2200	440	11	57	550	7700	440	2530	1100
Nursoy (Wyeth)	20	68	Soy isolate	2.1	Safflower oil	3.6	Sucrose, Corn syrup	6.9	9	20	11	660	462	13	2750	440	9.9	60	737	1045	440	3300	1100
Pro-Sobee (Mead-Johnson)	20	68	Soy isolate	2.5	Soy oil	3.4	Sucrose, Dextrose, Maltose, Dextrins	6.8	17	20	13	825	550	13	1760	440	15.4	57	550	8800	440	3300	660
Soyalac (Loma-Linda)	20	68	Soy	2.1	Soy oil	3.8	Sucrose, Dextrose, Maltose, Dextrins	6.6	14	21	10	660	550	16.5	2200	440	5.5	66	550	8800	440	3300	660
CHO-Free (Syntex)	12	40	Soy isolate	1.8	Soy oil	3.5	None	0.02	17	24	10	935	715	11	2200	440	11	57	550	8800	440	3300	1100
CASEIN HYDROLYSATES																							
Nutramigen (Mead-Johnson)	20	68	Casein hydrolized	2.2	Corn oil	2.6	Sucrose, Arrowroot starch	8.6	14	18	14	660	495	13	1760	440	11	57	550	8800	440	3300	660
Pregestimil (Mead-Johnson)	20	68	Casein hydrolized	2.2	MCT, Corn oil	2.8	Glucose, Glucose polymers	8.8	14	18	14	660	440	13	2200	440	11	57	550	8800	440	3300	660
ELEMENTAL FORMULA																							
Vivonex (Eaton)	30	101	Crystalline amino acids	2.0	Safflower oil	0.15	Glucose	23.9	37	30	51	560	560	10	2778	222	17	33	830	11,100	1100	5600	940
MEAT FORMULAS																							
Meat base (Gerber)	20	68	Beef heart	2.8	Sesame, Beef fat	3.3	Sucrose, Tapioca starch	6.2	7.8	9.7	5.9	980	650	13.7	1740	460	6	59	600	7200	800	2000	1000

Index

[Page numbers in *italics* refer to figures; page numbers followed by *t* refer to tables.]

Abdominal epilepsy, 116
Abdominal pain, 46–47
 psychogenic, 116–117
Abetalipoproteinemia, 115
Acetonemia, 46
Acetonuria, 46
Acrodermatitis enteropathica, 119–120
Adenoids, 60
Adulterants, 16–17, 110
Age factor, 7
Airway obstruction, 60
Albuminuria, orthostatic, 70
Alcohol ingestion, 156
Allergens
 in cow's milk, 13–15
 in human milk, 154–158
 in differential diagnosis of cow's milk allergy, 109–110
Allergic tension-fatigue syndrome, 67–69
Alopecia, 64
Alpha-lactalbumin, 12t, 14, 15, 18, 19t, 25, 27
Amino acids, 144, 192t
Anaphylactic reaction, 34–35, 38t, 71
Anemia, 64–65
Angioedema, 62–63
 hereditary, 116
Antibacterial factors, 148t

Antibiotics, 17, 110
Antibodies
 in human milk, 147, 150
 to cow's milk proteins, 23–27, *24*
Antihistamines, 130–131
Anti-infective factors, 146–147, 148t
Antistaphylococcal factor, 151
Antiviral factors, 148t, 151
Appetite
 excessive, 85
 loss of, 52
Arrhythmias, 72–73
Arthus-like reaction; *See* Immune complex reaction
Aspiration, 118
Asthma, 55–56
Atopic dermatitis, 61–62
Aversion behavior, 52

B-cell dysfunction, 115
Beta-lactoglobulin, 11, 12t, 14–16, 18, 19t, 25, 27, 146
Beverages, milk-free, 176
Bifidus factor, 150
Bleeding, intestinal, 48–49, *50, 51*
Breast-feeding, 2, 5. *See also* Human milk

197

Breast-feeding *(continued)*
    advantages, 143–152
    adverse reactions, 154t
    immunologic advantages, 146–152
    infant problems, 153–154
    maternal advantages, 152
    maternal problems, 152–153
    nutritional advantages, 144–145
    in prevention, 143–158
    problems, 152–154
    promotion of, 162–163
    psychological advantages, 145–146
Bronchitis, 55

Caffeine, 156
Caffey's disease, 74
Calories
    in cow's milk, 13, 190t
    in human milk, 145, 190t
    in proprietary formulas, 195t, 196t
Candidiasis, 120
Carbohydrates, 12, 145
Cardiac arrhythmias, 72–73
Cardiovascular manifestations, 71–73
Caseins, 11, 12, 19t, 144
Celiac disease, 112, 115
Cell-mediated reaction, 34, 36–37, 38t
Central nervous system manifestations, 67–69
Challenge tests, 86–90
    oral challenge, 86–89, *87*
    subcutaneous provocation, 90
    sublingual provocation, 89–90
Chloridorrhea, congenital, 113
Cholesterol, 145
Cigarette smoking, 156
Colostrum, 146, 147, 149t, 151, 152
Commercial preparations, 13. *See also* Infant formulas
Complement, 27, 151
Complement-fixation test, 99
Condensed milk, 13
Congenital chloridorrhea, 113
Conjunctivitis, allergic, 74
Constipation, 52
Contact dermatitis, 63
Contact skin test, 91

Contamination, 16–17
Cookies, milk-free, 183–184
Coproantibodies, 98
Cor pulmonale, 72
Coronary heart disease, 72
Cortical hyperostosis, infantile, 74
Cough, 55
Cow's hair, 16
Cow's milk
    amino acids, 192t
    constituents, 11–22, 190–191t, 195t
    fatty acids, 193t
    processing, 17–19
Cow's milk allergy
    age at onset, 7
    diagnosis, 83–107
    differential diagnosis, 109–122
    as health problem, 5–6
    historical background, 1–3
    management, 123–136
    manifestations, 45–82
    pathogenesis, 23–44
    prevalence, 6–7t
    prognosis, 137–139
Cromolyn, 131–132
Cross-reactivity, 15–16
Cystic fibrosis, 112
Cystitis, 70
Cytotoxic food test, 100
Cytotoxic (cytolytic) reaction, 34

Death, sudden infant, 73–74
Delayed hypersensitivity. *See* Cell-mediated reaction
Dermatitis herpetiformis, 63–64
Dermatologic manifestations, 61–64, 62t
    differential diagnosis, 119–120
Desserts, milk-free, 185–187
Diarrhea, 47
Dichlorodiphenyl-trichloroethane (DDT), 157
Dieldrin, 157
Dietary management, 123–129, 161
    milk-free recipes, 129, 175–187
Disaccharides, 53
Drug antigens, human milk, 156–157
Disodium cromoglycate, 131–132

INDEX

Eczema, 61–62
Edema, oral, 52
Elimination diet, 125, 128
　for milk, 123–125
Enterocolitis, 49
Enterokinase deficiency, 113
Enteromammary immune system, 31, *32*
Enuresis, 69–70
Enviromental pollutants, 157–158
Enzymatic reactions, 2
Enzyme abnormalities, 52–54
Enzyme-linked immunosorbent assay (ELISA), 96
Eosinophilia, 67, 93
Epicutaneous tests, 90–91
Epidemiology, 5–9
Epilepsy, abdominal, 116
Erythroderma desquamativa, 119
Evaporated milk, 13, 18

Family history, 85–86
Fat, 12–13, 145
Fatty acids, 144, 193t
Fecal antibodies, 98
Fecal blood loss, 48–49, *50, 51*
Feeding practices, 110–111
Fluroescent immunosorbent test, 96
Food additives, 111
Food antigens, in human milk, 155
Food diary, 85
Food industry, 163–164
Food introduction, 161
Foreign substances, in cow's milk, 16–17, 110
Freezing, human milk, 159, 160t

Galactosemia, 113
Gamma globulin, 14, 15, 18, 19, 25
Gamma radiation, 19
Gastroenteritis, 114
Gastrointestinal manifestations, 46t, 46–54
　differential diagnosis, 110–117
Gastrointestinal protein loss, 49
Gastrointestinal tract transport, 28–31, *30*

Glue ears, 61
Gluten-induced enteropathy, 112
Goat's milk, 15–16, 129
　nutritional constituents, 195t
Gravy, milk-free, 182
Growth deficiency, 73

Hair, cow's, 16
Heat treatment, 17–19
　of cow's milk, 127–128
　of human milk, 158–159, 160t
Hemagglutination test, 99
Hematologic manifestations, 64–67
Hemosiderosis, 58–60, *59*
　pulmonary, 118–119
Heptachlorepoxide, 157
Hereditary angioedema, 116
Hexachlorobenzene, 157
Hexachlorocyclohexane, 157
Histamine release, 100
Homemade preparations, 129
Homogenization, 13
Human Lactation Center, Ltd., 162
Human milk, 129, 143
　allergens, 154–158
　aminoacids, 192t
　antibodies, 147, 150
　anti-infective factors, 146–147, 148t
　constituents, 190–191t, 195t
　cross-reactivity, 16
　drug antigens, 156–157
　environmental pollutants, 157–158
　fatty acids, 192, 193t
　food antigens, 155
　immunoglobulins, 147, 149t
　immunologic properties, 158–159, 160t
　nutritional advantages, 144–145
　pollutants, 154–158
　processing, 158–159, 160t
Human-milk banking, 158–159, 160t
Hydrolysates, 128
Hypoallergenic formulas, 159, 161, 164, 196t
Hypogammaglobulinemia, 115
Hypoproteinemia, 65
Hyposensitization, 132–133

Ichthyosis, 120
Immediate hypersensitivity. *See* Anaphylactic reaction
Immune complex reaction, 34, 35–36, 38t
Immune complex test, 99–100
Immune response
 in healthy person, 23–26, *24*
 in milk-sensitive subject, 26–27
Immune system, enteromammary, 31, *32*
Immunodeficiency disease, 115
Immunofluorescence studies, 53–54
Immunoglobulin A, secretory, 31–33, 61
Immunoglobulin E, (serum), 94
Immunoglobulins, 12t, 19t, *24–25*, 27
 human milk, 147, 149t, 158–159, 160t
Immunoglobulins (serum), 93–94
Immunology, 2, 33–37, 38t
 breast-feeding and, 146–152
Immunosorbent tests, 96
Infant death, 73–74
Infant diet, food introduction, 161
Infant formulas, 5, 13, 18, 126, 159, 161, 163–164, 195t, 196t
 advertisement for, 162, 163–164
 constituents, 195t, 196t
Infantile cortical hyperostosis, 74
Infectious rhinitis, 117
Injection hyposensitization, 133
Insect bites, 120
Insecticides, 157
International Council of Infant Food Industries, 164
Intestinal biopsy, 101
Intestinal bleeding, 48–49, *50, 51*
Intestinal lipodystrophy, 115
Intestinal lymphangiectasia, 114
Intestinal obstruction, 114
Intestinal parasites, 114
Intracutaneous tests, 90–91
Intrauterine sensitization, 27–28
Iron, 144, 145
Iron deficiency anemia, 64–65
Irritation rashes, 119

Keratitis, allergic, 74

Lactalbumin, 11, 12t
Lactoferrin, 149t, 150
Lactoperoxidase, 150
Lactose, 12, 14
Lactose intolerance, 111–112
La Leche League International, 162
Lead poisoning, 116
Leiner's disease, 119
Leukocyte histamine release, 100
Leukocytes, 151
Leukorrhea, 74
Lipodystrophy, intestinal, 115
Lymphangiectasia, intestinal, 114
Lymphoblast transformation test, 100–101
Lymphokine production, 101
Lyophilization, human milk, 159, 160t
Lysozyme, 149t, 150

Malabsorption syndromes, 47–48
Management, 123–136. *See also* Prevention
 dietary, 123–129, 161
 hyposensitization, 132–133
 pharmacologic agents, 130–132
 prophylactic medication, 130–132
 sequelae therapy, 130
 symptomatic therapy, 130
Meat-base formula, 129
Meat dishes, milk-free, 177–178
Methylmercury, 157
Milk elimination, 123–125
Milk-free recipes, 129, 175–187
Milk-induced syndrome with pulmonary disease, 56–58, *57*
Milk refusal, 52
Milk substitutes, 126–129, 159, 161
Minerals, 144, 145
Mitogenic factor, 151–152
Mucosal morphology, 52–54
Muramidase, 150

Nephrotic syndrome, 70–71

Ocular allergy, 74
Oral challenge, 86–89, *87*

INDEX

Oral-challenge passive-transfer test, 92–93
Oral edema, 52
Oral hyposensitization, 132
Orthostatic albuminuria, 70
Otitis media, serous (secretory), 60–61

Parasites, 114
Pasteurization, 13, 18
  human milk, 159, 160t
Patient history, 84–86
Penicillin, 17, 110
Perianal rash, 63
Pharmacologic agents, 130–132
Physical examination, 86
Plexiglass reservoirs, 97
Pneumonia, 56–58, 57
Pollutants, 110, 157–158
  human milk, 154–158
Polybrominated biphenyls (PBBs), 157–158
Polychlorinated biphenyls (PCBs), 157
Prausnitz-Küstner reaction, 92–93
Precipitation test, 96–98, 97
Prevention, 141–173
  breast-feeding in, 143–158
  human-milk banking in, 158–159, 160t
  milk substitutes in, 159, 161
  role of infant-food industry, 163–164
  role of medical profession, 161–162
  role of women's organizations, 162–163
  techniques, 142
Proctalgia, 52
Prostaglandin synthesis inhibition, 131
Protein, 11–12, 144, 145
Protein fractions, 12t, 18, 19t
Protein hydrolysates, 128
Protein loss, 49
Provocation tests, 89–90
Psychogenic abdominal pain, 116–117
Pulmonary disease, 56–60, 57, 59
Pulmonary hemosiderosis, 58–60, 59, 118–119
Purpura, 63

Radioallergosorbent test (RAST), 94–95
Recipes, milk-free, 175–187
Respiratory manifestations, 54t–61
  differential diagnosis, 117–119
Respiratory tract obstruction, 60
Rhinitis, 54–55
  nonallergic, 117

Salad dressings, milk-free, 180
Salads, milk-free, 181
Sauces, milk-free, 182
Seborrhea, 63, 119
Secretory immunoglobulin A, 31–33, 61
Serum albumin, 12t, 14, 15, 19t, 25
Sex factor, 7, 8t
Sheep's milk, 16
Shwachman syndrome, 112
Skim milk, 13
Skin tests, 90–93
  contact, 91
  epicutaneous, 90–91
  intracutaneous, 90–91
  Prausnitz-Küstner passive transfer test, 92–93
  skin window, 91–92
Skin window, 91–92
Soybean formulas, 126–127, 161
Steatorrhea, 47
Stomatitis, 52
Subcutaneous provocation, 90
Sublingual hyposensitization, 133
Sublingual provocation, 89–90
Sucrose intolerance, 113
Sudden infant death syndrome, 73–74

T-cell dysfunction, 115
Tension-fatigue syndrome (allergic), 67–69
Terminology, 2
Tests and testing, 86–101
  for anaphylactic reaction, 35
  challenge tests, 87–90
  intestinal biopsy, 101
  skin tests, 90–93
  in virto tests, 93–101

Theophylline, in human milk, 156
Thriving failure, 73
Thrombocytopenia, 65–67, *66*, 115
Thyroid hormones, in human milk, 145
Tonsils, 60
Trypsin digests, 19
Tuberculin reaction, in breast-fed infants, 151

Ulcerative colitis, 51–52, 113
Ultraviolet radiation of cow's milk, 19
Urinary manifestations, 69–71
Urologic disorders, 116
Urticaria, 62

Vasomotor rhinitis, 117
Vegetable diets, 129
Vegetable dishes, milk-free, 179
Villous atrophy, 53
Vomiting, 46

Wheezing, 117–118
Whey proteins, 11, 12t, 144
Whipple's disease, 115
White snakeroot, 110
Wiskott-Aldrich syndrome, 115
Wolman's disease, 115
Women's organizations, 162–163

Zinc deficiency, 120